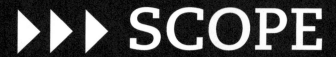 **SCOPE**

Special Children's Outreach and Prehospital Education

Authors

Terry A. Adirim, MD, MPH
Interim Director
Pediatric Emergency Medicine
St. Christopher's Hospital for Children
Associate Professor of Emergency Medicine
  and Pediatrics
Drexel University College of Medicine
Philadelphia, Pennsylvania

Elizabeth "Betsy" Smith, CFRN, NREMT-P
AirCare Flight Nurse
PHI Air Medical Group Northeast
Weyer's Cave, Virginia

Primary Contributor
Tasmeen Singh, MPH, NREMT-P
Center for Prehospital Pediatrics
Children's National Medical Center
Washington, DC

JONES AND BARTLETT PUBLISHERS

Sudbury, Massachusetts

BOSTON   TORONTO   LONDON   SINGAPORE

Jones and Bartlett Publishers
World Headquarters
40 Tall Pine Drive
Sudbury, MA 01776
978-443-5000
info@jbpub.com
www.jbpub.com

Jones and Bartlett's books and products are available through most bookstores and online booksellers. To contact Jones and Bartlett Publishers directly, call 800-832-0034, fax 978-443-8000, or visit our website, www.jbpub.com.

Substantial discounts on bulk quantities of Jones and Bartlett's publications are available to corporations, professional associations, and other qualified organizations. For details and specific discount information, contact the special sales department at Jones and Bartlett via the above contact information or send an e-mail to specialsales@jbpub.com.

Some images in this book feature models. These models do not necessarily endorse, represent, or participate in the activities represented in the images.

Notice: The patients described in the case studies throughout this text are fictitious.

ISBN-13: 978-0-7637-2468-9
ISBN-10: 0-7637-2468-8

Production Credits

Chief Executive Officer: Clayton E. Jones
Chief Operating Officer: Donald W. Jones, Jr.
President, Higher Education and Professional Publishing: Robert W. Holland, Jr.
V.P., Sales and Marketing: William J. Kane
V.P., Production and Design: Anne Spencer
V.P., Manufacturing and Inventory Control: Therese Connell
Publisher, Public Safety Group: Kimberly Brophy
Editor: Jennifer L. Reed
Production Editor: Susan Schultz
Photo Researcher: Christine McKeen
Director of Marketing: Alisha Weisman
Text Design: Anne Spencer
Cover Design: Kristin Ohlin
Composition: NK Graphics
Text Printing and Binding: Courier

Additional credits appear on page 107, which constitutes a continuation of the copyright page.

Library of Congress Cataloging-in-Publication Data
Adirim, Terry.
  Special children's outreach and prehospital education (SCOPE) / Terry Adirim, Elizabeth Smith, and Tasmeen Singh.
    p. ; cm.
  Includes bibliographical references.
  ISBN 0-7637-2468-8 (pbk.)
  1. Pediatric emergencies—Handbooks, manuals, etc. 2. Children with disabilities—Medical care—Handbooks, manuals, etc.
  [DNLM: 1. Emergency Treatment—Child—Handbooks. 2. Child, Exceptional—Handbooks. 3. Disabled Children—Handbooks. 4. Emergency Medical Services—Child—Handbooks. WS 39 A235s 2006] I. Smith, Elizabeth, 1962- II. Singh, Tasmeen. III. Title.

RJ370.A324 2006
362.4'083—dc22
                                2005018127

6048

Printed in the United States of America
18 17 16 15 14   10 9 8 7 6 5

Contents

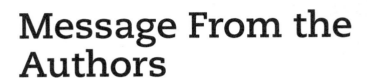

Message From the Authors

Early one morning on my very first day as an attending physician in a pediatric emergency department, my very first patient was a little girl presenting in respiratory distress and shock. She was 5 years of age, but appeared to be the size of a 6-month-old child. Her mother stated that she had a genetic syndrome that "even Johns Hopkins couldn't figure out." The emergency room (ER) team immediately went to work. We manually ventilated the child. We searched for a place on her arms and legs to put a peripheral IV line. X-rays were taken, medications given, and IV fluid boluses initiated. We diagnosed the child with a perforated bowel and soon she was on her way to the operating room.

The child's mother remained calm during the entire episode and we largely ignored her during the resuscitation except when we periodically asked her pertinent questions about the child's medical history. As soon as we finished our work, I turned to the child's mother. I realized that the triage nurse had brought the child back to the treatment room—not prehospital providers. I asked the mother how her child was transported to our ER. The child's mother told me that she drove from home. Shocked, I asked her, "How long did it take for you to get here?" She stated that it was a 2-hour drive. Even more surprised, I asked her why she did not call 9-1-1. Her answer became my inspiration for *SCOPE*. She said that she did not trust prehospital providers to know how to treat her child and worse, they would take her to the community hospital where "she surely would have died."

Despite the fact that children with special health care needs (CSHCN) are a small subset of the pediatric population, these children account for a significant proportion of emergency department visits and ambulance transports. Pediatric tertiary care centers most often serve as home hospitals for these children and are prepared to provide the complicated care that these children need. However, most children are cared for in general emergency departments and by emergency medical services that have little experience in the care of medically complicated children. Because most of these children live at home with their families, their parents and caregivers necessarily become experts in their care. The purpose of *SCOPE* is to educate prehospital providers and nonpediatric emergency providers in the emergency care of CSHCN so that the medical provider as well as the families of CSHCN can be more confident in the emergency care that these children receive.

We dedicate this program to CSHCN and their families who inspire us and to the thousands of caring prehospital providers who have taken a SCOPE course and who have helped to shape the final program.

Terry Adirim, MD, MPH

Emergency Medical Services and Children with Special Health Care Needs

Twelve million children in the United States have special health care needs. Children with special health care needs (CSHCN) are those who have, or are at risk for, chronic physical, developmental, behavioral, or emotional conditions and who also require health and related services of a type or amount not usually required by typically developing children.[1] Advances in medical science and technology have been instrumental in allowing children with complex medical problems to survive beyond the neonatal period. Moreover, family-centered care has been the goal for the care of these children and so many of these children are living in our communities as opposed to living in institutions. These children are frequent users of the emergency medical system.

Children with special health care needs are usually in the care of adults who have been trained to manage their child's daily care. In general, families are knowledgeable about their child's technology and medical conditions. Families may have detailed medical plans that specify the size of tubes, how often to change tubes, dosages of medications, ventilator settings, etc.

Emergency medical services (EMS) is mainly activated during the time of a crisis. This crisis may occur because of equipment failure or because of a panicked caregiver who is fatigued or new to caring for the child. Sudden respiratory distress or arrest will invariably prompt a call for help.

A survey of 100 families with CSHCN conducted at Children's National Medical Center (CNMC) demonstrated that although 97% of the families had sought emergency care in the past, only 23% of the caregivers had ever called 9-1-1 before, while 93% had driven their child to the hospital during an emergency. There are several reasons why parents choose not to call 9-1-1. The CNMC survey showed that 30% of the parents/care-givers were afraid that their children would be transported to the nearest community hospital and not taken to the hospital where they normally received care. Ten percent of the caregivers did not trust the care that emergency responders could provide and 36% of the parents felt that they could transport their children more rapidly by driving them directly to their home hospital.

CSHCN often have multiple medical problems. These can include underlying neurological disorders as well as developmental delays and mental retardation. Some children have sensory deficits such as blindness and hearing loss. CSHCN may be smaller than other children their age and depending on their underlying medical condition, CSHCN may have vital signs that differ from the norms for age. These issues need to be taken into consideration when caring for these children. Parents are often able to give this information to emergency providers. Many children have emergency information forms or medical jewelry where this information is accessible.

Since children with special health care needs often present with uncommon medical conditions that are unfamiliar to emergency responders, the purpose of this program is to improve the prehospital care responder's knowledge and comfort level with chronically ill and technology dependant children. The purpose of this student manual is to provide basic information on various chronic medical conditions these children may have, as well as on technologies and equipment that may be necessary for their survival. Ultimately, the goal is to educate the EMS community in how to care for and manage children with special health care needs in the event of a medical or traumatic crisis.

[1] McPhearson M, Arango P, Fox H, et al. A new definition of children with special health care needs. *Pediatrics*. 1998;102:137–140

Prehospital Notification Programs

Prehospital notification programs are beneficial for both prehospital providers and families of children with complex medical problems. Even though caregivers and families of chronically ill and/or technology dependent children complete specialized training, they may encounter a crisis that requires EMS intervention. Therefore, families, in conjunction with the child's health care team, are encouraged to develop an emergency care plan to predetermine interventions that should be taken during an emergency. Prehospital notification programs exist sporadically in various jurisdictions in the United States. Components of such programs typically include notification letters to local emergency services (fire and EMS) that describe the child's medical problems and suggest medical management. These notification letters provide prehospital responders with the opportunity to learn about CSHCN in their service area and familiarize themselves with the children that have uncommon illnesses or specialized technology. Families also benefit from this program, as they are comforted knowing that EMS is aware of their child's medical issues.

In 1999, the American Academy of Pediatrics (AAP) in collaboration with the American College of Emergency Physicians (ACEP) developed an emergency department notification program. A child's primary pediatrician completes a two-page medical information form called an Emergency Information Form (EIF) that is then carried by the child's caregivers. The form also allows the child to be enrolled into the MedicAlert program, which keeps the child's medical information in a database that is accessible by phone 24 hours a day, 7 days a week, to medical providers directly responsible for the emergency care of the child.

In 1999, Children's National Medical Center (CNMC) in Washington, DC developed its own version of a prehospital notification program that eventually enrolled over 700 children. The program, called "EMS Outreach," was designed to inform local EMS about CSHCN in the ambulance service's immediate response area. Families of CSHCN cared for at CNMC are given the opportunity to enroll their child into this program. Caregivers are given a packet of information that describes the EMS system and addresses transportation destinations and other issues that may arise in an emergency situation. The packet also reminds caregivers to call their local electric and phone company so that the utilities may be prenotified of the child's issues so that when there are any scheduled power outages, the CSHCN receives priority for return of service or notified when unexpected power outages will continue for a prolonged period of time. This gives caregivers time to search for an alternative method to power their child's medical equipment.

The importance of the EMS Outreach program was demonstrated in a survey of prehospital providers conducted at CNMC. This survey of over 700 emergency responders in the Washington DC area showed that only 22% of providers who have treated CSHCN in the past were comfortable with the treatment and care that they provided for the child. Ninety percent of the providers who had received a medical information form found the form useful.[1]

Like with the AAP/ACEP program, EMS Outreach enrollees complete a one-page medical information form. This form contains basic demographic and medical information about the child. The form also contains contact information for the child's primary caregiver and physicians. This medical information form is faxed to a predesignated representative of the child's local EMS jurisdiction who forwards the information to the EMS providers stationed closest to the child's address. This information is also entered into the respective jurisdiction's 9-1-1 dispatch system provided that technology is available in the area.

When providers receive medical information forms through programs such as EMS Outreach, they are encouraged to review the information received and familiarize themselves with the child's medical conditions. For complicated cases, providers are encouraged to call families and arrange to make home visits. Home visits give providers the opportunity to meet the child, to become familiar with specialized home equipment and any technologies the child may require for survival, to identify potential hazardous materials (i.e., oxygen tanks and compressors) and to establish a relationship with the family. During this time, complicated issues such as the choice of hospital destinations in an emergency or a child's Do Not Resuscitate (DNR) order can be discussed. Such prenotification measures better prepare EMS providers to handle potentially complex emergencies and increase knowledge levels so that the prehospital provider can confidently care for children with special health care needs. The CNMC prehospital provider survey showed that 93% of prehospital providers who had conducted a home visit benefited from the visit.

When conducting a home visit, the following check list may be helpful to prehospital providers to ensure a productive visit:

- Call the caregivers and arrange a mutually convenient time and place to meet.
- Assess any language barriers with the child or his/her caregivers.
- Familiarize yourself with the child's developmental age and level of understanding.
- Familiarize yourself with the child and his/her technologies and/or home health care equipment.
- Review fire safety plans with the caregivers and child.
- Discuss transportation issues, including mode of transport and the location of transport, in the event of an emergency.
- Address any questions about the child's medical conditions, medications, or allergies.
- Arrange an interval where you may want to follow up with the caregiver for updates on the child's conditions.
- Educate the caregiver about your 9-1-1 system setup and when and how to access help in the event of an emergency.

[1] Adirim T, Singh T, Smith E, Tuanquin L, Wright J. Survey of Prehospital Provider Knowledge, Experience, and Comfort in the Care of Children with Special Health Care Needs, ABSTRACT, 2001 *Pediatric Academic Societies Meeting, May 2001.*

Acknowledgements

Other Contributors:
Craig Engler, RRT
Genny Gebus, RN
Anne Conway, PT
Vicky Freedenberg, PNP
Mamata Kamat, MBBS, MPH

Veronica LeMay, RN
Carolyn Ramwell, PNP
Sarah Storing, RN
Kathy Wiggins, RN

We would like to thank the District of Columbia Fire/EMS Department, Montgomery County EMS (Montgomery County, Maryland), and Fairfax County Fire and Rescue Department (Fairfax County, Virginia) for supporting the program. Their feedback has been instrumental in the development of SCOPE.

We would like to thank the following individuals for their support and encouragement:
Jane Ball, RN, PhD
Wayne Neal, RN
Bob Waddell, NREMT-P
Milree Williams
Emergency Medical Services for Children Program

The original SCOPE program was funded by a grant from EMSC/MCHB/HRSA.

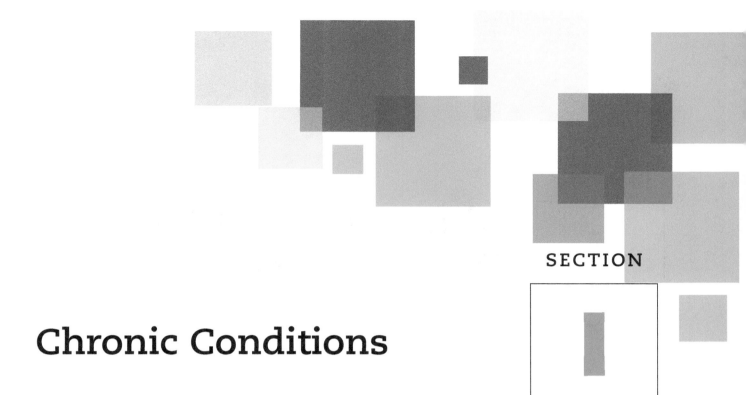

SECTION

I

Chronic Conditions

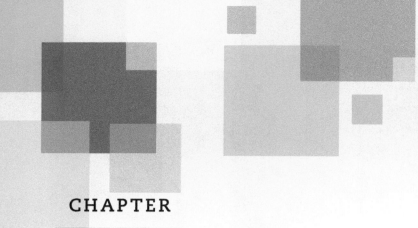

CHAPTER

1 Pulmonary Disorders and Airway Defects in Children

▶▶▶ case presentation

Jenny is a 6-year-old girl who sustained a brain stem injury after removal of a brain tumor at age 4. Since then, she has a depressed respiratory drive and is mechanically ventilated through a tracheostomy tube. Her caregiver called 9-1-1 because Jenny developed sudden onset of respiratory distress. The caregiver suctioned the tracheostomy tube, but there was no relief of the distress.

1. When EMS arrives, what should be the first intervention?
2. What are the most common causes of Jenny's problem?

▼ case progression

Upon arrival, EMS notes that Jenny is having difficulty breathing despite being on the ventilator. She is removed from the ventilator and manual ventilations with a bag-mask device are initiated. It is noted that she is difficult to ventilate. Preparations for a tracheostomy tube change are made while her caregiver suctions the existing tracheostomy tube. Another tracheostomy tube is found in Jenny's "go bag." After suctioning twice, it is noted that she is still having difficulty breathing. However, after the tracheostomy tube change it is much easier to ventilate her manually. A large mucous plug in the old tube is noted. Jenny and her caregiver are prepared for transport to their home hospital.

Apnea

Sleep apnea is defined as a lapse of spontaneous breathing during sleep. It is a cessation in breathing for more than 20 seconds or one that is associated with a change in color, limpness, altered mental status or bradycardia (**Figure 1-1**). Apnea occurs more frequently in infants born prematurely and generally reflects immature neurologic and respiratory control mechanisms.[1]

Pauses in respiration may be due to central apnea, which is a condition where there is an absence of a neurologic signal from the brain to the respiratory muscles. The cause can be due to disorders such as encephalitis, brain stem infarction, or tumor, or it can be congenital or idiopathic. Neuromuscular disorders such as muscular dystrophy or thoracic restrictive disorders such as kyphoscoliosis[2] can cause weakness of the respiratory muscles that leads to ineffective respirations. Often these children will eventually need mechanical ventilation as their condition deteriorates.

A common type of obstructive apnea in infants is due to gastroesophogeal reflux (GER). This is when the stomach contents reflux up the esophagus and into the

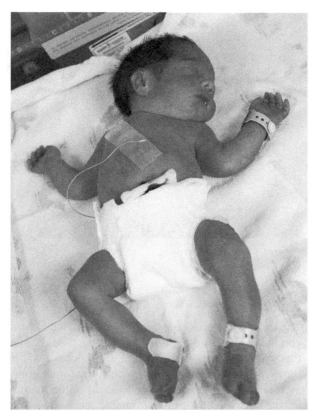

Figure 1-1 Sleep apnea.

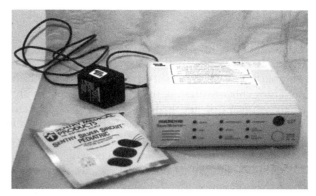

Figure 1-2 Home apnea monitor.

airway. Most children can be treated medically and will outgrow this condition. The most common type of childhood apnea[2] is obstructive sleep apnea that occurs due to an occlusion in the upper airway at the oropharyngeal level. This can be seen in children with markedly enlarged tonsils and adenoids or in very obese children where the tissues of the upper airway are redundant and therefore block the airway when these tissues are relaxed during sleep. Mixed apnea, often seen in premature infants, is central apnea and obstructive apnea. Often this is due to prematurity of the brain centers that control respirations together with GER.

Signs and Symptoms

- Altered level of consciousness (ALOC)
- Poor respiratory effort
- Cyanosis
- Limpness
- Bradycardia
- Respiratory and/or cardiac arrest

Treatment

Obstructive sleep apnea may be managed by providing continuous positive air pressure (CPAP) during sleep that is delivered through a nose mask or tra-

cheostomy tube. Central apnea is sometimes managed with supplemental oxygen or medications that stimulate the respiratory system or if severe, through mechanical ventilation. A child diagnosed with sleep apnea may be sent home with an apnea monitor to record his/her breathing patterns and alert parents and caregivers to an episode of apnea (Figure 1-2).

Prehospital Management

BLS and ALS Interventions

- Assessment and treatment of the ABCs
- Provision of supplemental oxygen (or manual resuscitation when indicated)
- Suction through the nose, mouth, or tracheostomy tube as needed
- Closely monitor the heart rate and respiratory rate of any infant experiencing apnea
- BLS—transport the patient on the apnea monitor
- ALS—transport the child on the apnea monitor, cardiac monitor, and pulse oximetry if available
- Follow PALS guidelines if the child is unresponsive and bradycardic, or if the child becomes pulseless or apneic

Home/Medical Management

- Apnea monitor
- Medications: anti-reflux, caffeine
- Tracheostomy tube and/or mechanical ventilator
- Continuous positive airway pressure (CPAP)

Apnea monitors should be transported with the child to the hospital. Most monitors contain a computer chip that records information that can be downloaded into a computer at the home hospital to determine the origin of the monitor alarms (high or low heart rate, apnea, or artifact). This diagnostic procedure can be expedited when the child is transported to his or her "home" hospital.

Asthma

Asthma is the most common chronic disease in children. It is an obstructive disease characterized by the narrowing of small airways due to inflammation and bronchoconstriction. In 1998, 3.8 million children 0 to 17 years of age had an asthma episode/attack resulting in 867,000 asthma-related ER visits and 174,000 hospitalizations. The ER visit rate is highest among children 0 to 4 years of age, with 170 visits per 10,000 children. Hospitalizations are also highest in this age group, with a hospitalization rate of 47 per 10,000. Among children, asthma deaths are rare. In 1998, 246 children 0 to 17 years of age died from asthma, or 0.4 deaths per 100,000 children compared with 2.6 deaths per 100,000 for adults 18 years of age and over.[1]

An asthma attack is an episodic event that may last from a few minutes to a few hours. A patient may experience an attack that lasts up to several weeks if left untreated. When serious symptoms persist, the patient is said to be in *status asthmaticus*. During an attack, there is an inflammatory response in the airways along with smooth muscle constriction that leads to narrowing of the airways. This creates the hallmark "wheeze" heard on auscultation. There can also be thick mucous secretions. Patient presentation will depend on the severity of an attack, which may range from mild to life-threatening. Factors that may trigger an asthma attack include infections, environmental allergens (such as smoke, molds, pollen, dust), animal dander, exposure to cold, and exercise.

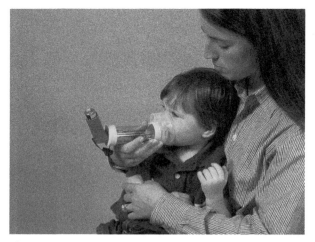

Figure 1-3 Asthma treatment.

Treatment

The treatment of an acute asthma attack includes bronchodilators and oral steroids (**Figure 1-3**). Bronchodilators act on the smooth muscle of the bronchioles of the lungs for temporary relief of asthma symptoms. Steroids are important to decrease the inflammation in the airways. Chronic or maintenance treatment sometimes includes inhaled steroids (e.g., Flovent) or inhaled chromolyn sodium (e.g., Intal) daily. Newer maintenance medications include Singulair, which is an oral medication, and Advair, a combination inhaled medication containing an inhaled steroid and a long-acting bronchodilator.

Signs and Symptoms

- Coughing
- Audible wheezing
- Tachycardia
- Tachypnea
- Dyspnea
- Use of accessory muscles

Prehospital Management

BLS Interventions
- Assessment and management of airway, breathing, and circulation
- Supplemental oxygen

ALS Interventions
- Nebulized albuterol
- Subcutaneous epinephrine (1:1000)

Home/Medical Management

- Aerochambers
- Nebulizer machines
- Peak flow meters
- Written asthma "action" plan
- Medications
  - Bronchodilators (e.g., albuterol, Xopenex)
  - Oral or inhaled anti-inflammatories (e.g., Vanceril, prednisone, Intal)
  - Anticholinergics (e.g., Atrovent)

Bronchopulmonary Dysplasia

Bronchopulmonary dysplasia (BPD) is a chronic lung disease occurring in infants that is characterized by stiff lungs and chronic lung disease. BPD is a worldwide problem with 5,000 to 10,000 new cases occurring each year and ranking with cystic fibrosis and asthma as the most common chronic lung disease in infants.[3]

BPD develops primarily in low birth weight infants who have respiratory distress syndrome (RDS), a lung disease common in premature babies. Babies born prior to 32 weeks gestation may not have enough surfactant to keep their alveoli (air sacs) open.[4] BPD may result from alveolar damage caused by lung disease, exposure to prolonged high oxygen concentrations, and mechanical ventilation after birth.[4]

A combination of fewer air sacs with a lack of surfactant can result in abnormally stiff lungs. This increases the work of breathing for affected infants who can quickly fatigue. As infants progressively weaken, carbon dioxide builds up in the lungs and blood. Respiratory infections can also worsen the inflammatory response in the lungs, leading to more fluid in the lungs and/or bronchospasm. Wheezing will result when tiny muscles in the bronchial tubes become narrower and spasm. In addition, air sacs soak up fluid from injured lung tissue, which results in lung stiffness and difficulty breathing. Other emergencies directly related to BPD include pulmonary edema, aspiration of food or stomach contents into the lungs, and apnea.

Signs and symptoms of BPD can vary in severity depending on the infant's lung maturity. They may include tachypnea, retractions, paradoxical respirations, abnormal posturing, and wheezing.

BPD causes the most difficulties during the first year of life, and most deaths from BPD also occur during this first year. Problems after the first year become increasingly uncommon. The most common long-term lung complication of BPD is asthma. Approximately one half of the children with BPD will have asthma. Other less common complications coexistent with BPD include apnea during infancy, gastroesophageal reflux, pulmonary hypertension, high blood pressure, pulmonary edema, aspiration, subglottic stenosis, and tracheomalacia. Infants who have BPD are at risk for frequent hospitalizations because of their borderline respiratory reserve, hyperactive airway, and increased susceptibility to respiratory infection. In the prehospital setting, EMS may be summoned to assist a baby with BPD who is experiencing respiratory distress.

Signs and Symptoms

- Increased respiratory rate
- Subcostal, intracostal retractions
- Increased oxygen requirement
- Paleness or cyanosis

Treatment

Home management of BPD may include oxygen, bronchodilators, corticosteroids, diuretics, antibiotics, and/or, in rare cases, ventilator support through a tracheostomy.

Home/Medical Management

- Reflux precautions
- Supplemental oxygen
- Antibiotics
- Diuretics
- Steroids
- Bronchodilators
- Nebulizer machine
- Tracheostomy (rare)
- Ventilator support (rare)

Prehospital Management

BLS Interventions
- Assessment and management of airway, breathing and circulation
- Oxygen

ALS Intervention
- Nebulized albuterol

Cystic Fibrosis

Cystic fibrosis (CF) is a genetic disorder that affects 30,000 Americans.[5] Progressive lung disease, pancreatic insufficiency, gastrointestinal obstruction, and an excess of sodium and chloride in the sweat are characteristic of CF. CF is an autosomal recessive disorder. The disease is caused by an aberrant protein that blocks the channel through which chloride enters and leaves the cell, resulting in the formation of thick viscous mucous.

The abnormal volume of thick mucous in the ducts of certain organs, such as the lungs, leads to life-threatening infections. Furthermore, thick secretions in the pancreatic ducts result in a smaller, thinner, and firmer pancreas. Pancreatic enzymes are unable to reach the duodenum, and therefore digestion and absorption of nutrients (fats, proteins, and carbohydrates) are markedly impaired. Because of the damage to the pancreas, some children develop diabetes mellitus. In the liver, focal biliary obstruction and fibrosis are common and may eventually lead to biliary cirrhosis. A few children develop hypertension, splenomegaly, ascites, and/or esophageal varices with gastrointestinal hemorrhage. The primary factor responsible for multiple clinical manifestations of the disease is mechanical obstruction caused by the increased viscosity of mucous gland secretions. However, pulmonary complications pose the most serious threat to life.[5]

Signs and symptoms of the disease vary with illness severity and may include chronic or persistent coughing, wheezing, recurring respiratory infections, respiratory distress, excessive appetite, hemoptysis (coughing of blood), and abdominal pain and discomfort. Additional complications can include dysrhythmias, cor pulmonale (enlargement of the right side of the heart), nasal polyps, clubbing of the hands and feet, pneumothorax, sinusitis, low weight gain/poor growth, rectal prolapse, and other disorders such as diabetes, liver and pancreatic diseases, and gall stones.

Signs and Symptoms

- Increased respiratory rate
- Subcostal, intracostal retractions
- Increased oxygen requirement
- Rales or wheezes on lung exam
- Paleness or cyanosis

Treatment

The current life expectancy of people with CF is approximately 30 years of age, whereas 50 years ago the maximum life expectancy was 5 years of age.[6] The treatment for cystic fibrosis is supportive and is aimed at preventing obstruction of the airways, enhancing mucous clearance in the lungs, and improving nutrition.

Symptomatic relief includes giving the active form of the abnormal protein product, chest therapy with bronchial or postural draining to reduce secretions, antibiotics to prevent and treat infections, and nutritional supplements to offset gastrointestinal complications. Pulmonary problems may be managed with oxygen and bronchodilators administered through nebulizer machines. Many children with CF require frequent hospitalizations, and they may closely resemble an adult patient with emphysema because of their thin, pale, barrel chest appearance.

Home/Medical Management

- Nebulizer machines
- Aerochambers
- Supplemental oxygen
- BiPAP or CPAP
- Vigorous chest physical therapy
- Chest physical therapy vest
- Central venous line
- Tracheostomy tube
- Medications
- Bronchodilators
- Enzyme replacement tablets
- Antibiotics

Prehospital Management

- Assessment and management of airway, breathing, and circulation
- Position of comfort
- Supplemental oxygen
- Nebulized albuterol

Tracheomalacia

Tracheomalacia is an abnormality of the tracheal walls causing them to be abnormally weak due to the loss of supporting cartilage and structural integrity, which frequently leads to a collapse of the trachea on inspiration. Tracheal collapse is most prominent during times of increased airflow, such as when the infant is coughing, crying, feeding, or has an upper respiratory infection. Causes of tracheomalacia can be congenital, extrinsic, or acquired. A congenital or intrinsic tracheal anomaly (occurring within the trachea) is a tracheoesophageal fistula (a patent connection between the trachea and esophagus); an extrinsic (occurring outside the trachea) anomaly includes defects such as abnormal development of the vasculature around the trachea that may create a ring, placing pressure on the trachea and interfering with airflow, and acquired malacia, which occurs in children with prolonged intubation or history of chronic tracheal infections.

Signs and Symptoms

- Coughing
- Prolonged expiratory phase
- Stridor
- Accessory muscle use
- Hypoxia
- Possible cyanosis
- History of chronic or recurrent pulmonary infections
- Respiratory arrest

Treatment

Medical management for tracheomalacia mostly consists of symptomatic treatment. A child with tracheomalacia may experience respiratory compromise with simple viral infections. Racemic epinephrine may decrease swelling of the upper airway under these circumstances. It is prudent to observe these children in hospital until they are no longer compromised. For children who have severe tracheomalacia, a stent, or a rigid piece of cartilage, may be surgically placed in the collapsed area of the trachea in order to establish permanent patency. Most children outgrow tracheomalacia. Infants with vascular rings may have constricting vessels surgically divided and reattached to surrounding structures in order to release the pressure on the trachea. In rare instances, a tracheostomy would be surgically placed in order to provide a patent airway until the child's airway grows and strengthens. Regardless of the underlying cause of tracheomalacia, infants and children in respiratory distress will present with similar signs and symptoms.

Home/Medical Management

- Positioning
- Supportive care

Prehospital Management

- Assessment and management of airway, breathing, and circulation
- Position of comfort
- Supplemental oxygen
- Nebulized epinephrine
- Subcutaneous epinephrine

◼ Tracheal Stenosis

Tracheal stenosis is a rare disorder that may be acquired or congenital, and is a contraction or narrowing of the lumen of the trachea. The most common type is acquired as a result of prolonged intubation, tracheostomy, a tumor, infection, or trauma. In comparison, congenital tracheal stenosis occurs when an area of the tracheal lumen narrows as a result of a cartilaginous tracheal ring abnormality. Children who have congenital tracheal stenosis often have associated anomalies of the respiratory tract, esophagus, skeleton, and heart.

Signs and Symptoms

- Coughing
- Wheezing
- Accessory muscle use
- Shortness of breath on exertion
- Stridor
- Hypoxia
- Possible cyanosis
- Croup
- Below normal pulse oximetry readings
- Possible history of recent intubation or **trachea decannulation**
- Recurring infections

Treatment

Management of these children includes endoscopic dilatation and anti-inflammatory medications on a short-term basis. Long-term management requires surgical repair ("cricoid split") or a tracheostomy.

Home/Medical Management

- Supplemental oxygen
- Tracheostomy management

Prehospital Management

- Assessment and management of airway, breathing, and circulation
- Position of comfort
- Supplemental oxygen
- Nebulized epinephrine

◼ Tracheal Atresia

Tracheal atresia is complete obstruction of the lumen of the trachea. The infant is born with an inability to breathe or ventilate. Until the obstruction can be surgically corrected, the child must have a tracheostomy placed. Respiratory distress can develop after surgical repair and decannulation of the tracheostomy tube as a result of scar tissue growth from the surgical suture lines in the tracheostomy.

Signs and Symptoms

- Increased respiratory rate
- Subcostal and intracostal retractions
- Increased oxygen requirement
- Paleness or cyanosis

Home/Medical Management

- Nebulizer machines
- Aerochambers
- Supplemental oxygen
- Apnea monitor
- Pulse oximeter monitor
- Suction machine
- Tracheostomy tube
- Mechanical ventilation
- Feeding catheter
- Feeding pump
- Medications
  - Bronchodilators
  - Oral or inhaled anti-inflammatory medications

Prehospital Management

BLS Interventions
- Assessment of airway, breathing, and circulation
- Humidified oxygen

ALS Interventions
- Nebulized albuterol or epinephrine
- Bag-mask ventilation of tracheostomy
- If there is still respiratory distress, even with manual ventilation, check for tracheostomy tube obstruction
- Suction tracheostomy tube
- If there is a tracheostomy obstruction, see tracheostomy section for tube change procedure

Potential Medical Emergencies

The most common medical problem encountered in a child who has a chronic pulmonary disease or a tracheal anomaly is respiratory compromise. Children with airway anomalies may have respiratory distress seemingly out of proportion to their acute problem, such as with an upper respiratory infection (URI). Children with tracheomalacia and a URI should be considered to have a compromised airway and transported to a hospital for evaluation and treatment. Children with chronic lung diseases such as BPD, asthma, or cystic fibrosis who are in respiratory distress should be assumed to have an infection or exacerbation of their underlying diseases. The cause of the respiratory compromise may differ with each underlying condition, but the emergency treatment of these conditions is similar. Assessment and management of the airway is always first. In a child with an airway anomaly, opening and positioning the airway may be the only maneuver necessary to relieve the compromise.

If the child is still in respiratory distress, administer oxygen. Consider bronchodilators in children with chronic lung diseases. Follow the respiratory rate and if available, assess pulse oximetry. If the child is still in respiratory distress and appears to be near respiratory failure or is in respiratory failure, then the child's ventilations need to be assisted either with bag-mask ventilation or through intubation of the airway with assisted ventilations.

Prehospital Management

BLS Interventions
- Assessment and management of the ABCs
- Place the child in a position of comfort
- Provide supplemental oxygen (or manual resuscitation when indicated)
- Suction through the nose, mouth, or tracheostomy tube as needed

ALS Interventions*
- Provide cool mist humidified oxygen to the child experiencing stridor
- Give a nebulized bronchodilator treatment for wheezing
- Administer nebulized 1:1000 epinephrine for severe stridor
- Administer SQ 1:1000 epinephrine 0.01mg/kg (0.01 cc/kg) to a maximum dose of 0.3 mg (cc) for a severe asthma attack
- Place the child on cardiac and pulse oximetry monitors if available
- Follow PALS guidelines if the patient's heart rate is less than 60, or if the patient becomes pulseless or apneic

*Follow local protocols or consult your medical control for appropriate drug administration

EMS Tips

Caring for Children With . . .

Chronic Respiratory Problems

1. If the child is over 6 years of age and has a peak flow meter at home, ask the child to blow into his or her flow meter to determine a current peak flow reading. If the child blows less than 50% of his or her "personal best" reading or is physically unable to blow into the meter, the child is in severe respiratory distress.

2. Ask the parent or caregiver if any medications were given to the child in the past 2 hours in an attempt to reverse respiratory distress. Monitor for therapeutic and adverse effects of these medications. Base further management and interventions on therapies already given at home.

3. If an infant receives home oxygen therapy of 2 L/min or less via nasal cannula and presents in respiratory distress, do not give more than 2 liters of oxygen through the nasal cannula. Instead, increase oxygen concentration delivery by providing blow-by oxygen or by placing a facemask at no less than 6 L/min over the child's nose and mouth.

4. Children who have cystic fibrosis often have a large, extremely expensive supply of medications in their home. Ask the parents if they want the medications transported to the hospital with the child.

5. Noxious exhaust fumes from an idling emergency vehicle can trigger bronchial spasm and worsen respiratory distress. Prevent inhalation of exhaust fumes when the child is outside the emergency vehicle. This can be accomplished by either briefly shutting down the engine or by giving oxygen or a nebulizer treatment by a facemask.

References

1. Wilson JD, Braunwald E, Isselbacher KJ, Petersdorf RG, Martin JB, Fauci AS, Root RK, eds. *Harrison's Principles of Internal Medicine*, 12th ed. New York, NY: McGraw-Hill.
2. National Center for Health Statistics. New asthma estimates: Tracking prevalence, health care, and mortality. 5 October, 2001. Available at: www.cdc.gov/nchs/products/pubs/pubd/hestats/asthma/asthma.htm. Accessed June 2004.
3. National Heart, Lung, and Blood Institute, National Institutes of Health. Bronchopulmonary dysplasia, NIH Publication No: 98-4081, November 1998. Available at: www.nhlbi.hih.gov/health/public/lung/other/bpd. Accessed June 2004.
4. Children's Hospital of Eastern Ontario. Bronchopulmonary dysplasia. Available at: http://www.cheo.on.ca/english/2012a.html. Accessed June 2004.
5. National Heart, Lung, and Blood Institute, National Institutes of Health. Facts about cystic fibrosis. Publication no: 95:3650, November 1995. Available at: www.nhlbi.nih.gov/health/public/lung/other/cystfib.htm. Accessed June 2004.
6. Cystic Fibrosis Foundation. Living with CF. Available at: www.cff.org. Accessed June 2004.

Resources

Cystic Fibrosis Foundation. Available at: www.cff.org. Accessed June 2004.

Medline Plus: Cystic fibrosis. Available at: http://www.nlm.nih.gov/medlineplus/cysticfibrosis.html. Accessed June 2004.

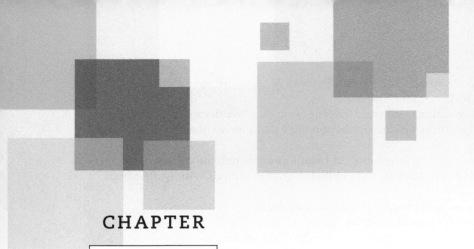

2 Cardiovascular Defects in Children

> ▶▶▶ **case presentation**
>
> Kayla is a 4-month-old infant born with tetrology of Fallot. Kayla's mother called 9-1-1 because she was concerned that Kayla was having difficulty breathing. When EMS arrives, they note a small infant in respiratory distress. Her vital signs are heart rate of 170 beats/min, respiratory rate of 70 breaths/min, and blood pressure of 90/60 mm Hg. Her pulse oximetry is 91% in room air.
>
> 1. What are the primary concerns?
> 2. How should the prehospital responder manage this patient?

> ▼ **case progression**
>
> EMS has assessed her airway, breathing, and circulation. They are appropriately concerned with her respiratory status. Kayla is immediately placed on a cardiorespiratory monitor and administered oxygen. Her mother states that Kayla has been sick for the last few days and has not been able to tolerate fluids by mouth. Also, she has vomited her cardiac medications. The EMS providers now suspect either an illness with impending cardiac failure or existing cardiac failure. IV access is obtained and Kayla prepared for transport to her home hospital.

Congenital Cardiovascular Defects

Congenital cardiovascular defects are among the most common forms of malformations in newborns. Incidence of congenital heart defects (CHD) estimated in different studies varies from 4/1000 to 50/1000 live births.[1] The diagnosis is established within the first year of life in 40% of patients with congenital heart disease.[2] Left untreated, many of these conditions prove fatal in most cases before age 20.[3] Cardiovascular defects are considered to be the leading cause of neonatal death due to congenital abnormalities despite an almost 40% decline in mortality from 1979 to 1997. This decline is due to advances in medical technology, early diagnosis, and better management over the last two decades.[4]

When an infant is born with a severe cardiac anomaly, palliative surgery is sometimes performed in the neonatal period and subsequent treatment is primarily directed towards home health care until definitive surgery can be performed. Depending on the abnormality, supportive care in the home is recommended when the defect cannot be surgically repaired.

Fetal Circulation

A connection between the right-sided pulmonary circulation and the left-sided systemic circulation is known as shunting. In the fetus there are four shunts: (1) placenta, which receives 55% of mixed (right and left ventricular) blood; (2) foramen ovale, a gap between the left and right atria; (3) ductus arteriosus, a channel between the pulmonary artery and the aorta; and (4) ductus venosus, a channel between the inferior vena cava and the placenta.[5] In the fetus only 15% of the blood goes through the lungs. The primary source of nutrient and gas exchange in the fetus is the placenta. After birth in the normal newborn, the placenta is separated from the newborn and there is a closure of the foramen ovale, ductus arteriosus, and ductus venosus. There is a simultaneous expansion of the lungs, which then functions as the center for exchange of gases.[5]

Congenital Heart Disease General Considerations

Signs and symptoms of congenital heart disease depend on the cardiac lesion. In general, developmentally these children are small for age. Many have an increased respiratory and heart rate. Those children with cyanotic heart disease will appear pale or bluish with baseline pulse oximeter readings in the low 80s. Many children with complex congenital heart disease can develop cardiac failure. The signs and symptoms of cardiac failure include:

- Increased respiratory rate
- Subcostal and intercostal retractions
- Tachycardia
- Heart murmurs
- Pallor
- Cyanosis
- Poor perfusion
- Delayed capillary refill
- Liver margin palpable below right costal margin
- Extremity edema
- Poor feeding and/or sweating with feeds

Home/Medical Management

- Monitors
- Oxygen
- Feeding tubes
- Digoxin
- Lasix

Treatment

Home treatment depends on the lesion and the severity of the condition. Children with lesions that cause heart failure may be on medications to control CHF such as digoxin and Lasix. Some children with cardiac defects do not grow well and may be on supplemental feedings either orally or through a feeding tube. Certain cardiac lesions require a palliative surgical procedure at birth and then a definitive surgical procedure later, or the definitive repair is performed as soon as the child is big enough to undergo surgery. The type of procedure is lesion dependent.

Prehospital Management

BLS Interventions
- Assessment and management of airway, breathing, and circulation
- Position of comfort
- Oxygen, do not go above child's baseline pulse oximetry

ALS Interventions
- If in respiratory failure, consider endotracheal intubation
- IV access
- IVF only if directed by medical control

Types of Defects

Acyanotic Defects

Acyanotic lesions account for the majority of congenital heart disease in newborns. In acyanotic defects there can be mixing of desaturated (poorly oxygenated venous) blood in the systemic arterial circulation, but the oxygen saturation is in the normal range. Many of these defects are associated with left-to-right shunts and obstruction to ventricular outflow. Left-to-right shunts cause oxygenated blood from the left side of the heart to mix with deoxygenated blood from the right side of the heart.

Some of the more common acyanotic cardiac defects include ventricular septal defects (VSD) and atrial septal defects (ASD). VSDs are holes in the lower chambers of the heart (**Figure 2-1**). The hole is most

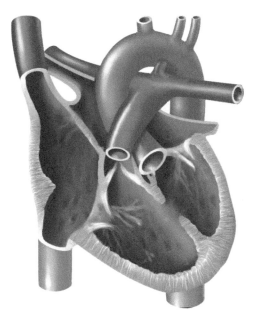

Figure 2-1 Image of a VSD lesion.

commonly through the muscle, but can sometimes also be in the membranous portion of the ventricle. Many of the holes in the muscular portion get smaller and eventually close. If the holes are large, then the child can have a left-to-right shunt and can develop congestive heart failure (CHF). These children may need medications to control their CHF and often will need surgery to close the hole. Note that children with large holes may not have murmurs on auscultation, and children with very small holes may have very loud murmurs. ASDs are holes in the upper chambers of the heart. Often, this condition is not diagnosed until the child is older than the infant age range. This condition may not cause symptoms until later in life but, when diagnosed, is often repaired surgically.[1]

Signs and Symptoms

- Acyanotic heart disease
- Increased respiratory rate
- Retractions
- Signs of heart failure, some of which include rales with lung exam, palpable liver edge, and swelling of the extremities

Patent Ductus Arteriosus

During development, fetal blood bypasses the lungs and is carried from the pulmonary artery to the descending aorta through a structure called the ductus arteriosus. After birth, a failure in the closure of this channel leads to the condition called patent ductus arteriosus (PDA). PDA represents 5% to 10% of all CHD.[5]

The disorder can occur in both premature and full-term infants. Clinical presentation depends on the size of the ductus arteriosus and is usually asymptomatic if the ductus is small. If the duct is large or if left untreated, the child may present with poor feeding, shortness of breath, recurrent infections, and CHF. Characteristic clinical findings include increased heart rate, heart murmur, and/or a bounding pulse.

Signs and Symptoms

- Increased respiratory rate
- Subcostal and/or intracostal retractions
- Poor feeding
- Extremity edema
- Tachycardia
- Holosystolic heart murmur

Treatment

In premature infants, an attempt is made to close the PDA by fluid restriction and prostaglandin inhibitors such as indomethacin. Surgical ligation (tying) of the

PDA is undertaken if medical management does not close the ductus. In full-term infants, surgical ligation of the patent ductus is indicated if heart failure develops. If the infant is asymptomatic, surgery may be postponed until 6 months to 3 years of age or until problems develop. Surgical treatment is associated with a very low risk of complications, and prognosis is good after surgery.

Home/Medical Management

- Cardiorespiratory monitor
- Oxygen (rarely)
- Medications such as Lasix
- Feeding tubes

Prehospital Management

BLS Interventions
- Assessment and management of airway, breathing, and circulation
- Position of comfort
- Oxygen
- Transport to home facility if local protocols allow it

ALS Interventions
- Cardiorespiratory monitor
- If respiratory failure, consider endotracheal intubation
- Intravenous access
- Intravenous fluid only with medical control permission

Atrial Septal Defect

Atrial septal defect (ASD) is a defect in the septum that separates the upper two chambers of the heart, the atria, and accounts for 5% to 10% of all congenital heart defects.[5] Infants and children with this defect are usually asymptomatic. When the defect is small there is a very high rate of spontaneous closure and, hence, surgical correction is delayed until the child is 3 to 4 years of age. However, if the defect is large and/or left untreated, the patient may present with congestive heart failure or pulmonary hypertension, which may be irreversible and may be fatal.

Signs and Symptoms

- Increased respiratory rate
- Subcostal and/or intracostal retractions
- Extremity edema
- Poor feeding
- Rales on lung exam
- Liver palpable below costal margin
- Tachycardia
- Fixed split S2 on cardiac exam (late in course)

Treatment

Children with isolated ASDs are surgically repaired. This procedure is usually performed by a pediatric cardiovascular surgeon at a tertiary care center. If left unrepaired, the child can develop CHF with fluid overload to the lungs. This can lead to pulmonary hypertension that is eventually fatal.

Home/Medical Management

- Usually none, as most young children are asymptomatic

Prehospital Management

BLS Interventions
- Assessment and management of airway, breathing and circulation
- Oxygen
- Position of comfort
- Transport to home hospital if local protocols allow it

ALS Interventions
- If in respiratory failure, consider endotracheal intubation
- Cardiorespiratory monitoring
- Intravenous access
- Intravenous fluids if recommended by medical control

Ventricular Septal Defect

Ventricular septal defect (VSD) is a defect where there is failure of adequate development of the cardiac wall separating the two lower chambers of the heart, the ventricles. The defect can be in the muscular part of the ventricular wall or the membranous portion. VSDs are the most common congenital heart disorder and occur in nearly 15% to 20% of all children with CHD.[5] This defect is sometimes associated with other congenital heart defects.

Signs and Symptoms

If in congestive heart failure:
- Increased respiratory rate
- Subcostal and/or intracostal retractions
- Rales on lung exam
- Poor feeding and/or sweating with feeding
- Extremity edema
- Increased heart rate
- Systolic heart murmur
- Liver edge palpable below the right costal margin

Treatment

Smaller defects are usually asymptomatic and often close on their own. At times an audible murmur can be appreciated. Patients with larger defects often present with difficulty feeding, growth and developmental delay, recurrent infections of the respiratory tract, and congestive heart failure. Open-heart surgery is the most common choice of treatment. Prior to the closure of these defects, the child is at risk of developing endocarditis, which is prevented by prophylactic measures, such as antibiotics.

Home/Medical Management

- Feeding tubes
- Medications such as digoxin and Lasix

Prehospital Management

BLS Interventions
- Assessment and management of airway, breathing, and circulation
- Oxygen
- Position of comfort
- Transport to home hospital if local protocols allow it

ALS Interventions
- If in respiratory failure, consider endotracheal intubation
- Intravenous access
- Intravenous fluid and/or medication as per medical control

Atrioventricular Canal Defect

Atrioventricular (AV) canal defect (endocardial cushion defect or atrioventricular septal defect) is a defect between the atrium and ventricles of the heart. The tricuspid and mitral valves abnormally form into one single valve, allowing oxygenated blood from the left side of the heart to enter the right side, mixing with venous blood. Nearly 40% of heart defects in patients with Down syndrome are atrioventricular canal defects.[5]

Signs and Symptoms

- This condition can lead to CHF
- Increased respiratory rate
- Subcostal and/or intracostal retractions
- Rales on lung exam
- Poor feeding and/or sweating with feeding
- Extremity edema
- Increased heart rate
- Systolic heart murmur
- Liver edge palpable below the right costal margin

Most infants with an AV canal defect have a delay in growth and are undernourished. Recurrent pulmonary infections and episodes of CHF are common symptoms presenting anytime from birth to several months of age.

Treatment

This defect is corrected with single or multiple surgeries. Some children are corrected soon after birth while others are not. Treatment of those children not corrected early may include medications to control CHF, such as digoxin and Lasix. Children with this defect may not grow well and often will be on supplemental feedings through feeding tubes.

Home/Medical Management

- Cardiorespiratory monitor
- Feeding tubes
- Medications such as Lasix and digoxin

Prehospital Management

BLS Interventions
- Assessment and management of airway, breathing, and circulation
- Oxygen
- Position of comfort
- Transport to home hospital if local protocols allow it

ALS Interventions
- If in respiratory failure, consider endotracheal intubation
- Intravenous access
- Intravenous fluid and/or medication as per medical control

Obstructive Lesions

Obstructive lesions are lesions that produce obstruction to the ventricular outflow tracts. Some examples include pulmonary stenosis, aortic stenosis, and coarctation of the aorta.

Pulmonary Stenosis

The pulmonary valve is situated between the right ventricle and the pulmonary artery and allows blood to flow from the right ventricle to the lungs. An abnormality in the development of this valve leads to narrowing of the valve due to thickening or obstruction by abnormal muscle, a condition known as pulmonary stenosis (PS). PS accounts for 8% to 12% of all CHD.[5]

Infants may present with cyanosis if the stenosis is severe. However, most infants present with a mild condition and are usually asymptomatic. If the pulmonary stenosis progresses, right ventricular failure can occur. Symptoms of progressive stenosis include

shortness of breath and fatigue. Patient may present with hepatomegaly if the condition progresses to CHF.

Signs and Symptoms

- Respiratory distress
  - Increased respiratory rate
  - Subcostal and intracostal retractions
- Rales on lung exam
- Decreased feeding and/or sweating with feeds
- Poor growth
- Increased heart rate
- Liver edge palpable below costal margin
- Extremity edema

Treatment

If the right ventricular pressure becomes too high, the stenosis must be corrected. This can be done by a balloon valvuloplasty procedure during cardiac catheterization. Balloon valvuloplasty stretches the narrowed area of the valve allowing more flow of blood. If this procedure fails, patients require surgery to relieve the stenosis.

Home/Medical Management

- Supplemental oxygen (rarely)
- Medications to prevent CHF such as Lasix and digoxin

Prehospital Management

BLS Interventions
- Assessment and management of airway, breathing, and circulation
- Oxygen
- Position of comfort
- Transport to home hospital if local protocols allow

ALS Interventions
- If in respiratory failure, consider endotracheal intubation
- Intravenous access
- Intravenous fluid and/or medication as per medical control

Aortic Stenosis

Aortic stenosis is a malformation of the aortic valve. The aortic valve is situated between the left ventricle and the aorta. Specifically, the defect is the lack of one or two of the normal three leaflets (or cusps) of the valve. The remaining leaflets are thick and stiff.

Signs and symptoms depend on the severity of the condition. Most children are asymptomatic even though mild stenosis can worsen over time. Presentation is usually in adulthood. Severe stenosis can occur in childhood. Symptoms of worsening stenosis can include fatigue, dizziness, fainting, and chest pain.

Signs and Symptoms

- Fatigue
- Dizziness
- Fainting
- Poor feeding
- Chest pain
- Systolic heart murmur

Treatment

A balloon valvuloplasty can stretch the narrowed area. If surgery is performed, the valve is replaced and may still work in a mildly abnormal way, causing the patient to limit some types of exercise. Follow-up care requires prophylaxis for prevention of infection.

Home/Medical Management

- Antibiotic prophylaxis for invasive medical procedures

Prehospital Management

BLS Interventions
- Assessment and management of airway, breathing, and circulation
- Oxygen
- Position of comfort
- Transport to home hospital if local protocols allow it

ALS Interventions
- If in respiratory failure, consider endotracheal intubation
- Intravenous access
- Intravenous fluid and/or medication as per medical control

Coarctation of the Aorta

Coarctation of the aorta is a condition where there is a constriction of the aorta. The aorta is the great artery supplying the body with oxygenated blood pumped from the left ventricle of the heart. Coarctation of the aorta represents 8% to 10% of all CHD. It is commonly associated with Turner syndrome, a genetic defect affecting girls.[5]

At birth the child is often asymptomatic. However, signs of coarctation can develop as early as a week after delivery if the defect is a critical coarctation of the aorta. Symptoms begin when the ductus arteriosus closes during the first week of life because there is then no way to bypass the obstruction in the aorta

to get oxygenated blood to the body. Symptoms include poor feeding, breathlessness, and signs of circulatory shock. Patients may present with weak peripheral pulses (especially in the left upper extremity and the lower extremities if the coarct is prior to the brachial artery), higher blood pressure readings in the upper extremities than in the lower extremities, or congestive heart failure.

Signs and Symptoms

- Poor feeding
- Respiratory distress including increased respiratory rate and retractions
- Increased heart rate
- Decreased peripheral pulses
- Systolic heart murmur
- Cool extremities
- Poor capillary refill

Treatment

Initially the problem is fixed surgically by either removing the stenosed segment or by placing a patch over the affected area. In the rare event that the problem recurs, it can be treated with a balloon angioplasty.

Home/Medical Management

- Cardiorespiratory monitors
- Feeding tubes

Prehospital Management

BLS Interventions
- Assessment and management of airway, breathing, and circulation
- Oxygen
- Position of comfort
- Transport to home hospital if local protocols allow

ALS Interventions
- If in respiratory failure, consider endotracheal intubation
- Intravenous access
- Intravenous fluid and/or medication as per medical control

Cyanotic Defects

These conditions occur when blood from the arteries and the veins mix in the heart, causing a constant low blood oxygen concentration. Typical pulse oximetry readings for children with uncorrected cyanotic heart lesions can range from the upper 70% range to the low 90%. The degree of cyanosis may vary with age, activity, or both. In many instances survivability depends on the presence of an opening between the right-sided pulmonary circulation and the left-sided systemic circulation. This concept is called shunting. This shunting allows unoxygenated blood to mix with oxygenated blood. During fetal life, two normal openings in the fetal heart allow this mixing of blood: (1) the foramen ovale (FO), a hole between the left and right atria, and (2) the ductus arteriosus (DA), a channel between the pulmonary artery and the aorta. However, the FO and DA usually close in healthy newborns between a couple of hours to several days after birth. Two openings that allow this mixing to occur after birth are other cardiac abnormalities: atrial septal defect (ASD) and ventricular septal defect (VSD). Acidosis is common and can develop quickly because of decreased ventilatory reserve. Medical practitioners should use supplemental oxygen with care in those babies who depend on a patent ductus arteriosus for the mixing. This is because oxygen promotes closure of the ductus. This type of heart disease can result in a true life-threatening emergency, since circulatory collapse is imminent after the development of acidosis. Some of the more common cyanotic cardiac defects include hypoplastic left heart syndrome, tetrology of Fallot, and transposition of the great arteries.

Hypoplastic Left Heart Syndrome

Hypoplastic left heart syndrome (HLHS) is characterized by inadequate development of the left ventricle and aorta and stenosis or atresia of the aortic and/or mitral valve. HLHS accounts for 9% of all newborn congenital heart defects[5] and is the most common cause of death during the first month of life due to congenital heart disease.

In this condition, the left side of the heart is unable to carry out its normal function of maintaining circulation throughout the body. The right side of the heart is therefore overworked to maintain both pulmonary (lung) and systemic (body) circulation. Infants with this defect develop profound systemic shock, hypoxemia, and cyanosis after the closure of the FO and DA, in the absence of a VSD or ASD. Emergent treatment involves administration of a medication, prostaglandin E_1, to reopen the DA; vasopressors, such as dopamine, and fluids to maintain cardiac output; as well as maintenance of airway and breathing through intubation and ventilation with oxygen. Correction of metabolic acidosis may also be necessary.[5]

Exogenous administration of oxygen can be harmful for infants with HLHS. Too much oxygen will dilate the pulmonary bed causing blood to flood the lungs and preventing its return to the body. Allowing carbon dioxide in the bloodstream to increase is beneficial. These children are mechanically ventilated on room air. A combination of acidosis with an increase of PA_{CO_2} levels in the 55 to 65 mm Hg range and hypoventilation resulting in oxygen saturation levels in the 70% range decreases pulmonary blood flow, which is desirable.

Signs and Symptoms

- Cyanosis
- Respiratory distress including increased respiratory rate and retractions
- Poor feeding
- Rales (crackles) on lung exam
- Poor perfusion including delayed capillary refill and decreased peripheral pulses
- Increased heart rate
- Decreased blood pressure
- Heart murmurs

Treatment

Infants born with HLHS have surgery soon after birth. However, the definitive surgical procedures are not performed until the child is older. The first surgery allows mixing of blood so that the child will get some oxygenated blood to the rest of his body. This is called a palliative procedure and is also called step one of the Norwood procedure. Many children with HLHS then typically have two more surgeries to repair the condition, a Hemi-Fontan and then, if indicated, the full Fontan procedures. Some families opt for heart transplantation. Between surgeries, these children are on medications such as digoxin and Lasix and may also be on supplemental feedings.

Home/Medical Management

- Cardiopulmonary monitor
- Feeding tubes
- Supplemental oxygen
- Medications including digoxin and Lasix

Prehospital Management

BLS Interventions
- Assessment and management of airway, breathing, and circulation
- Oxygen
- Position of comfort
- Transport to home hospital if local protocols allow it

ALS Interventions
- If in respiratory failure, consider endotracheal intubation
- Intravenous access
- Intravenous fluid and/or medication as per medical control

Tetralogy of Fallot

Tetralogy of Fallot (TOF) is the most common cause of congenital cyanotic heart disease in infants, representing 10% of all CHD[5] (Figure 2-2). There is a higher incidence of tetralogy of Fallot among children with Down syndrome. The original description of TOF included four different defects, hence the name *tetrology*: ventricular septal defect; obstruction of the right ventricular outflow tract; right ventricular hypertrophy (RVH); and overriding of the aorta. However, only two of the conditions are required to describe the condition: a large VSD and right ventricular outflow obstruction. RVH is considered to be a result of the ventricular outflow obstruction and the overriding of the aorta varies.[5]

Symptoms appear at birth or very soon afterwards. Newborns can be very cyanotic and are only able to survive if there are other associated cardiac defects that allow oxygenated blood to reach the body. The severity of the symptoms depends upon the type of associated defect and the resulting amount of oxygenated blood supplied to the general circulation. These children can experience sudden, severe periods of cyanosis with tachypnea and even unconsciousness. Older children may become short of breath or faint during periods of strenuous activity. These symptoms, more commonly referred to as "tet spells," occur due to a sudden lack of blood flowing to the lungs, resulting in decreased oxygenation.

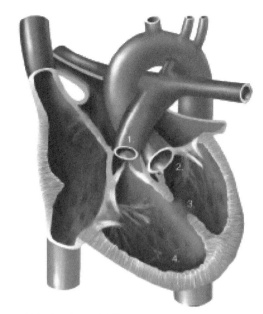

Figure 2-2 Tetralogy of Fallot.

Signs and Symptoms

- Respiratory distress including increased respiratory rate, retractions
- Cyanosis
- "Tet spell" with possible loss of consciousness
- Increased heart rate
- Decreased perfusion

Treatment

Treatment for a "tet spell" includes maneuvers that increase pulmonary blood flow. Infants and young children can be placed into a knee–chest position to increase systemic resistance. Management of the child includes use of morphine to suppress the respiratory center, control of acidosis using sodium bicarbonate, and fluids to increase systemic pressure. Oxygen benefits are limited since pulmonary blood flow is obstructed.[5] Infants with severe tetralogy of Fallot may need surgery to temporarily increase blood flow to the lungs by placing a shunt between the aorta and the pulmonary artery. This increase in perfusion to the lungs will result in improved oxygenation. Ultimately, the child will require open-heart surgery to repair many of the defects. The long-term results are usually good, but greatly depend on the severity of the defects.

Home/Medical Management

- Cardiorespiratory monitor
- Supplemental oxygen (rarely)
- Feeding tubes

Prehospital Management

BLS Interventions
- Assessment and management of airway, breathing, and circulation
- Oxygen
- Position of comfort
- If in a "tet spell," then put child in knee–chest position
- Transport to home hospital if local protocols allow it

ALS Interventions
- If in respiratory failure, consider endotracheal intubation
- Intravenous access
- Intravenous fluid and/or medication as per medical control

Transposition of the Great Arteries

Transposition of the great arteries (TGA) is a condition where there is a reversal of the pulmonary artery with the aorta such that the circulatory system is then a parallel circuit instead of a series circuit. The pulmonary artery normally carries venous blood from the right ventricle to the lungs, and the aorta normally carries oxygenated blood from the left ventricle of the heart to the body. In TGA, unoxygenated blood flows from the body to the right side of the heart through the aorta to the body again, while oxygenated blood flows from the lungs to the left side and back to the lungs again. TGA occurs in about 5% of all congenital heart defects.[5] If there is no other associated lesion, such as a ventricular septal defect that allows mixing of unoxygenated with oxygenated blood, then the infant can die.

Signs and Symptoms

- Cyanosis
- Respiratory distress including increased respiratory rate and retractions
- Respiratory arrest
- Increased heart rate
- Decreased blood pressure
- Poor perfusion
- Decreased peripheral pulses

Treatment

Newborns are extremely cyanotic and are only able to survive if there is another defect present to allow oxygenated blood to reach the body. Such defects may include ASD, VSD, or PDA. Immediate enlarging of the atrial opening using balloon arterial septostomy will reduce cyanosis and improve oxygenation. Ultimately, the child will need a definitive surgical procedure to correct this problem. The procedure is called an arterial switch. Simply, the aorta and pulmonary artery are disconnected and reconnected to their correct ventricles. Most infants do very well with this procedure. If left untreated, 90% of children die before the age of 6 months.[5]

Home/Medical Management

- Cardiorespiratory monitor
- Feeding tubes
- Central venous lines
- Supplemental oxygen
- Medications

Prehospital Management

BLS Interventions
- Assessment and management of airway, breathing, and circulation
- Oxygen
- Position of comfort
- Transport to home hospital if local protocols allow it

ALS Interventions
- If in respiratory failure, consider endotracheal intubation
- Intravenous access
- Intravenous fluid and/or medication as per medical control

Tricuspid Atresia

Tricuspid atresia is the absence of the tricuspid valve. It is one of the least common types of congenital heart disease, accounting for 1% to 3% of all CHD.[5] Due to the absence of the tricuspid valve, blood cannot flow from the right atrium to the right ventricle. This results in an underdeveloped and small right ventricle. This condition is further classified depending on the presence or absence of other defects such as pulmonary stenosis and TGA.

Signs and Symptoms

- Cyanosis
- Poor feeding
- Increased respiratory rate
- Retractions
- Increased heart rate
- Poor perfusion
- Decreased blood pressure

Treatment

The patient will present with severe cyanosis, which is usually present since birth. Other features include poor feeding habits and tachypnea. Survivability depends on whether an ASD or VSD is present. Cyanosis can be reduced by surgically placing a shunt to increase blood flow to the pulmonary circulation. There are other types of surgeries to repair or improve the problems associated with this defect.

Home/Medical Management

- Cardiorespiratory monitor
- Feeding tubes
- Central venous lines
- Supplemental oxygen
- Medications

Prehospital Management

BLS Interventions
- Assessment and management of airway, breathing, and circulation
- Oxygen
- Position of comfort
- Transport to home hospital if local protocols allow it

ALS Interventions
- If in respiratory failure, consider endotracheal intubation
- Intravenous access
- Intravenous fluid and/or medication as per medical control

Pulmonary Atresia

Pulmonary atresia is the absence of the pulmonary valve. The result is an inability for blood to flow from the right ventricle into the pulmonary artery and to the lungs. The right ventricle and tricuspid valve are underdeveloped. Pulmonary atresia occurs in about 1% of all children with CHD.[5] The presenting findings are cyanosis and tachypnea. Acidosis is common and can develop quickly because of decreased ventilatory reserve.

Signs and Symptoms

- Cyanosis
- Poor feeding
- Increased respiratory rate
- Retractions
- Increased heart rate
- Poor perfusion
- Decreased blood pressure

Treatment

Management of the condition is to keep patency of the ductus arteriosus using prostaglandins, cardiac catheterization, and urgent surgical procedures. Success of surgical repair is dependent on the severity of the defect. If condition left untreated the infant will die within 6 months of age in 85% of cases.[5]

Home/Medical Management

- Feeding tubes
- Central venous lines
- Supplemental oxygen
- Medications

Prehospital Management

BLS Interventions
- Assessment and management of airway, breathing, and circulation
- Oxygen
- Position of comfort
- Transport to home hospital if local protocols allow it

ALS Interventions
- If in respiratory failure, consider endotracheal intubation
- Intravenous access
- Intravenous fluid and/or medication as per medical control

Truncus Arteriosus

Truncus arteriosus is characterized by a single arterial trunk supplying pulmonary (lung), coronary (heart), and systemic (body) circulation. The result is one large arterial "trunk." A large VSD is always present along with a truncus defect, essentially making the right and left ventricles into a single chamber. Truncus arteriosus occurs in less than 1% of all children with CHD.[5] The infant is cyanotic since birth. Other features include poor feeding associated with dyspnea, recurrent pulmonary infections, and failure to thrive.

Signs and Symptoms

- Cyanosis
- Poor feeding
- Increased respiratory rate
- Retractions
- Increased heart rate
- Poor perfusion
- Decreased blood pressure

Treatment

In order to survive, surgery must be done early in life. Repair would include closing a large VSD, detaching the pulmonary arteries from the large common artery, and connecting the pulmonary arteries to the right ventricle with a graft. The condition is associated with mortality rate greater than 50%.[5]

Home/Medical Management

- Feeding tubes
- Central venous lines
- Supplemental oxygen
- Medications

Prehospital Management

BLS Interventions
- Assessment and management of airway, breathing, and circulation
- Oxygen
- Position of comfort
- Transport to home hospital if local protocols allow it

ALS Interventions
- If in respiratory failure, consider endotracheal intubation
- Intravenous access
- Intravenous fluid and/or medication as per medical control

Cardiac Arrhythmias

Cardiac arrhythmias, or an irregular heartbeat, may occur at any age. Some causes of arrhythmias in pediatrics include cardiac anomalies, certain over-the-counter medications, and electrolyte abnormalities. Often there is no recognizable cause of an arrhythmia. The child may be asymptomatic or may experience dizziness, lightheadedness, weakness, chest discomfort, nausea, irregular heartbeats, or fainting spells.

Types of Abnormal Pediatric Heart Rhythms

Sinus arrhythmia is characterized by cyclic changes in the heart rate during breathing. This is a normal finding in children and does not cause hemodynamic compromise. Sinus tachycardia occurs when the sinus node sends out electrical signals faster than usual, speeding up the heart rate. Some of the causes for sinus tachycardia (a heart rate less than 200 beats/min) include fever, crying, pain, shock, exercise, anemia, circulatory shock, CHF, allergic reaction, and fear. Supraventricular tachycardia (SVT) is a series of early beats in the atria that speeds up the heart rate (usually 240 ± 40 beats/min in infants, > 180 beats/min in older children). This arrhythmia is the most common abnormal tachyarrhythmia in children.[5] One common cause of SVT is Wolff-Parkinson-White (WPW) syndrome. WPW is an abnormal electrical pathway that exists between the atria and ventricles that causes the electrical signal to arrive at the ventricles too soon and is transmitted back into the atria. Very fast heart rates may develop as the electrical activity ricochets between the atria and ventricles.

Ventricular tachycardia (VT) is a condition where the heart beats fast due to electrical signals arising from the ventricles rather than from the atria. It is an uncommon pediatric arrhythmia, yet it is a potentially life-threatening condition. Causes of VT include serious heart disease, long QT syndrome, medications (such as anti-arrhythmic drugs, theophylline, cocaine, tricyclic antidepressants), and electrolyte imbalance. A very slow heart rate (< 80 beats/min in infants, < 60 beats/min in children) is called bradycardia. The most common cause of bradycardia is hypoxia. Other causes are hypothermia, hyperkalemia, hypothyroidism, and use of drugs such as digitalis. Sick sinus syndrome is a condition where the sinus node does not fire its signals properly, so the heart rate slows down. Sometimes the rate alternates between a slow and fast rate. This arrhythmia may be seen in some children who have had open-heart surgery. This condition is rare in children.

Treatment

Treatment depends on the condition. Some children with prolonged QT syndromes are on medications. Children with prolonged QT syndromes that lead to ventricular arrhythmias may have implanted pacemakers and cardiac defibrillators. Children with SVT may be on medications such as beta blockers. Children with previous cardiac surgeries may be at risk for sick sinus syndrome and may need pacemakers.

Home/Medical Management

- Cardiorespiratory monitor
- Feeding tubes
- Pacemakers
- Implanted cardiac defibrillators (ICD)
- Medications (e.g., propranolol, anticoagulation drugs such as Coumadin)

Prehospital Management

BLS Interventions
- Assessment and management of airway, breathing, and circulation
- Oxygen
- Position of comfort
- Defibrillation with automatic external defibrillators
- Transport to home hospital if local protocols allow it

ALS Interventions
- If in respiratory failure, consider endotracheal intubation
- Intravenous access
- Intravenous fluid and/or medication as per medical control (e.g., lidocaine)
- Defibrillation of ventricular tachyarrhythmias

Signs and Symptoms

- Dizziness
- Lightheadedness
- Weakness
- Chest discomfort, pain
- Nausea and vomiting
- Palpitations
- Fainting spells
- Congestive heart failure (respiratory distress, rales on lung exam, poor perfusion, poor feeding, extremity edema, liver edge palpable below costal margin)

Summary of Cardiac Defects in Children

Acyanotic defects are those lesions where there is no mixing of poorly oxygenated blood with oxygenated blood and the child's baseline color is pink. These lesions are the most common cardiac lesions and are usually found during a routine medical exam either during the neonatal period or when the child is older. Often only a murmur is heard. The severity of symptoms depends on the severity of the defect.

With cyanotic defects, blood from veins and arteries mix in the heart. There are low blood oxygen levels and in fact the child's baseline color may be blue. These lesions are less common than the acyanotic defects and are most often diagnosed within the first few days of life as the ductus arteriosus closes. Acidosis is a common problem due to decreased ventilatory reserve.

Home/Medical Management

- Supplemental oxygen
- Feeding catheters
- Internal pacemaker
- Medications
  - Diuretics
  - Anticoagulants
  - Antiarrthmics
  - Vasopressors
- Feeding pumps
- Pulse oximetry
- Internal defibrillator

Potential Medical Emergencies

Children with cardiac defects may present with one or more of the following: dyspnea, tachypnea, cyanosis, tissue hypoxia, bradycardia, congestive heart failure, irregular heart rhythms, and arrest. Approach these children as you would any other child by first evaluating the airway, breathing, and circulation. Open the child's airway and position the child. Assess respiratory rate and obtain pulse oximetry (**Figure 2-3**). Ask the caregiver for the child's usual pulse oximetry reading. For those children with cyanotic heart lesions, use oxygen only if the pulse oximetry reading is below the child's baseline, and then only administer enough to keep the child at his or her baseline pulse oximetry reading. Take care with the administration of fluids. If the child is in shock, you can bolus with normal saline. However, be aware that excess fluids can cause CHF. It is prudent to discuss fluid management with medical control.

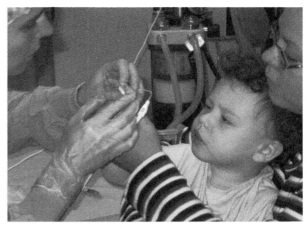

Figure 2-3 Obtain pulse oximetry reading.

Prehospital Management

BLS Interventions

- Assess and manage the ABCs
- Provide supplemental oxygen (use manual resuscitation if indicated)—use extreme caution in administering oxygen to babies who are "normally" blue (see earlier section, "Cyanotic Defects")
- Assess the cardiac rhythm (place on cardiac monitor if available)

ALS Interventions

- Establish IV access
- Consider IV Lasix 1 mg/kg if rales are present and child is already on Lasix
- Consider a 20 cc/kg normal saline IV fluid bolus (use caution if child is in CHF)
- Treat symptomatic cardiac arrhythmias, following PALS guidelines and local protocols (including the use of electrical therapy and medications)
- Avoid placing defibrillator/pacing pads or paddles over the internal pacemaker generator (usually found in the upper chest area); doing so can cause severe burns
- Consider the use of inotropes (dobutamine, dopamine) with severe hypotension, which is unresolved with fluid boluses
- Access medical control for these complicated patients and consider transporting to their home hospital. Always follow local EMS protocols with regard to transport and treatment protocols.

Caring for Children With . . .

Cardiac Defects

1. Ask the caregiver for the child's normal color and room air pulse oximeter reading. If the child normally has a bluish color or if the child's normal pulse oximeter readings are below 90%, **use extreme caution in providing supplemental oxygen**. Give enough supplemental oxygen to return the child to his or her normal baseline. Too much oxygen (which decreases CO_2) will dilate the pulmonary bed, allowing blood to flood the lungs and thus rob the body of blood flow. If the child remains on room air, lower CO_2 levels will cause the pulmonary bed to constrict and allow for better systemic perfusion.

2. If the child is on an anticoagulant medication such as Coumadin, use caution when starting an IV or when handling the child. These children can easily bruise and may have difficulty clotting. They follow "bleeding precaution" guidelines, since their medication keeps their clotting times below normal. They may use a home-monitoring device called a CoaguChek® monitor to track their therapeutic blood levels of the anticoagulation medication they are taking.

3. Any child who has recently undergone open-heart surgery for repair of a cardiac defect is at a higher risk for developing congestive heart failure several weeks to several months after hospital discharge. These children may be on a short-term course of Lasix in the post-operative period.

References

1. Hoffman JI, Kaplan S. The incidence of congenital heart disease. *J Am Coll Cardiol*. 2002;39:1890–900.
2. Moller JH, Allen HD, Clark EB, Dajani AS, Golden A, Hayman LL, Lauer RM, Marmer EL, McAnulty JH, Oparil S, Strauss AW, Tarbert KA, Wagner A. Special Report: Report of the Task Force on Children and Youth. American Heart Association 1993;88:2479–2486.
3. Cohen AJ, Tamir A, Houri S, Abegaz B, Gilad E, Omohkdion S, Zabeeda D, Khazin V, Ciubotaru A, Schachner A. Save a child's heart: We can and we should. *Ann Thorac Surg*. 2001;71:407–408.
4. Boneva RS, Botto LD, Moore CA, Yang Q, Correa A, Erickson JD. Mortality associated with congenital heart defects in the United States: Trends and racial disparities, 1979–1997. *Circulation*. 2001;103:2376–2381.
5. Park MK, Troxler GR. *Pediatric Cardiology for Practitioners*, 4th ed. St. Louis, MO: Mosby Yearbook; 2002:93–263.

Resources

Jaimovich D, Vidyasagar D. *Handbook of Pediatric and Neonatal Transport Medicine*. Philadelphia, PA: Hanley & Belfus; 1996;7:85–156.

McPhearson M, Arango P, Fox H, Lauver C, McManus M, Newacheck PW, Perrin JM, Shonkoff JP, Strickland B. A new definition of children with special health care needs. *Pediatrics*. 1998;102:137–140.

American Heart Association. Congenital cardiovascular disease. In: Heart and Stroke A–Z Guide, American Heart Association. Available at: www.americanheart.org/presenter.jhtml?identifier100 00056. Accessed June 2004.

Congenital Heart Information Network. http://www.tchin.org. Accessed February 16, 2004.

Medline Plus: Congenital Heart Disease. http://www.nlm.nih.gov/medlineplus/congenitalheartdisease.html. Accessed June 2004.

Down Syndrome

Jesse is a 3-month-old boy born with trisomy 21. His caregiver reports that he has been eating less and seems more lethargic than usual. This morning, his caregiver notes that he is breathing fast. She calls 9-1-1. When EMS arrives, they find a floppy baby in respiratory distress. He is pale and listless. His caregiver reports that he was born with a "heart problem."

1. What should be the first step?
2. What congenital conditions are associated with Down syndrome that could account for this baby's presentation?
3. What associated features of Down syndrome can be contributing to this child's condition?

▼ case progression

Upon encountering this child, EMS immediately assesses his airway, breathing, and circulation, and places him on a cardiorespiratory monitor. His airway is patent, his respiratory rate is 70 breaths/min and his heart rate is 180 beats/min. His perfusion is poor and he appears cyanotic centrally. Oxygen is given to achieve saturations in the 90s. Crackles on lung exam are noted and the EMS responders proceed to attempt placement of an IV. Also on exam EMS notes that the liver is about 4 cm below the right costal margin. IV access is accomplished on the third attempt. As EMS is working to stabilize this child, the caregiver gives them an information card that says that Jesse has a complete AV canal heart defect and is on digoxin and Lasix. EMS places a heplock on the IV and calls medical control for medication instructions. Medical control instructs the crew to give Lasix via IV and to transport the baby to his home hospital. Of note, children with Down syndrome often have floppy airways and large tongues that can worsen respiratory distress by causing airway obstruction.

▪▪ Down Syndrome

Down syndrome affects 1 in 800 births. This rate is lower than in the 1970s as a result of prenatal diagnosis and termination. The risk of Down syndrome (DS) increases with maternal age; however, the highest incidence is in women in their twenties.[1] Down syndrome is a specific complex of symptoms associated with mental retardation caused by chromosomal abnormalities.

There are three known types of chromosomal abnormalities that can lead to DS: translocation, mosaicism, and trisomy 21 (the most common). From a clinical standpoint, there isn't much difference between the translocation and trisomy 21 types, but there is an average of a 10- to 30-point higher IQ and fewer medical complications in the children with mosaicism. People with Down syndrome can be expected to live well into adulthood and the majority live in private or group homes (**Figure 3-1**).

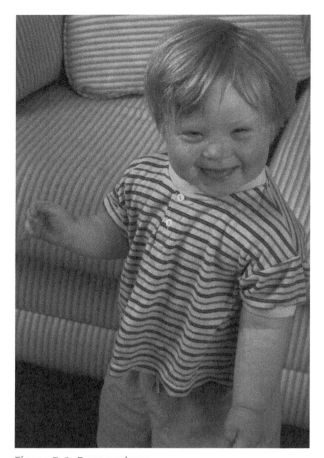

Figure 3-1 Down syndrome.

Table 3-1 Features and Common Conditions of Children with Down Syndrome	
Physical Features	**Common Conditions**
Large tongue	Congenital heart disease
Short neck	Orthopedic conditions
Obesity	Dental problems
Short stature	Seizures
Loose ligaments	Developmental delays
Epicanthal folds of eyes	

Children with DS are at increased risk of medical complications. Some of the organ systems affected include: cardiovascular, sensory, endocrine, orthopedic, dental, gastrointestinal, neurologic developmental, and hematologic. People with DS are developmentally delayed. They have IQs in the mentally retarded range and are commonly short in stature and overweight. Also, people with DS have anatomic differences that can impact on their emergency treatment.

People with DS have facial features and body habitus that are stereotypical for DS. Their eyes have epicanthal folds and are wide-set. They have a short neck. Their limbs and fingers are short, and they have a palmar crease (Table 3-1).

Medical Problems in Down Syndrome

Congenital Heart Disease

Two thirds of children born with DS have congenital heart disease, the most common being endocardial cushion defects (e.g., AV canal), ventricular septal defects, and atrial septal defects. The endocardial cushion is a connection between the atria and ventricles of the heart. Children born with this form of heart disease, AV canal, need surgery soon after birth, as uncorrected defects lead to heart failure and death. Many of these children with uncorrected congenital heart disease will appear blue because of the shunting of blood through the defect and the mixing of unoxygenated with oxygenated blood. Supplemental oxygen is unlikely to help under these circumstances. Often, postoperative patients with DS may have residual cardiac problems including pulmonary hypertension, cardiac failure, and conduction problems.

Emergency treatment of these children should include airway management, supplemental oxygen, and IV access. In patients with heart failure, diuretics should be considered with judicious fluid resuscitation only if necessary. (See Chapter 2, *Cardiovascular Defects in Children* for more details on management.)

Airway and Respiratory Problems

People with DS have large tongues and small oral and nasal cavities. This may make intubation more difficult than in children without DS. They also have malocclusions and other dental anomalies (abnormal contact of the upper and lower teeth). Tooth eruption tends to be later than usual. The enlarged tongue and dental anomalies can lead to speech abnormalities as well. In an emergency situation, if airway management is necessary, mask ventilation and intubation can be difficult. In the case of airway obstruction, a simple jaw thrust maneuver may be all that is needed to clear the airway. In an unconscious patient, either jaw thrust or a nasopharyngeal (NP) airway may be necessary. The NP airway diameter should be smaller than expected because of the smaller nasal passages. Approximately 25% of people with Down syndrome have tracheal stenosis.[2] This may have an impact on the choice of endotracheal tube size, so having tubes available that are one to two sizes smaller than expected is recommended.

Orthopedic Issues

Orthopedic conditions are common in children with DS. Most of the problems are due to ligamentous laxity (loose ligaments). Approximately 15% of children with DS have atlantoaxial subluxation, but only 1% become symptomatic and this rarely causes paralysis.[1] Atlantoaxial subluxation is when the ligaments of the cervical spine are so lax that they allow the first cervical spine to partially dislocate at the atlantoaxial joint. Symptoms related to atlantoaxial subluxation include: difficulty walking, abnormal gait, neck pain, torticollis, urinary incontinence, clumsiness, and spasticity. Other orthopedic problems include hip dislocation, patellar dislocation, and flat feet. Children with DS tend to be "floppy," so gross motor skills such as walking tend to be delayed.

Neurologic Conditions

A higher proportion of children with DS have epilepsy. Most of the seizures are of the generalized tonic-clonic type. Management is the same as with other children with seizures. Management of the airway, administration of oxygen, and IV access are important emergency maneuvers.

EMS Tips

Caring for Children With . . .

Down Syndrome

1. Children with DS may have airway compromise when unconscious.
2. Peripheral IV access may be more difficult than usual because these children tend to be overweight.
3. These children are developmentally delayed, so they may not be able to give you an accurate history of their medical problems.

References

1. Roizen NJ. Down syndrome, In: *Children with Disabilities*, 5th ed. Batshaw ML, ed. Baltimore, MD: Brookes Publishing Company; 2002.
2. Greenberg JA, Shannon MT. Down syndrome: implications for emergency care. *JEMS* 1995;20:39–51.

Resources

National Down Syndrome Society. Available at: http://www.ndss.org. Accessed June 2004.

National Association for Down Syndrome. Available at: http://www.nads.org. Accessed June 2004.

Medline Plus: Down Syndrome. Available at: http://www.nlm.nih.gov/medlineplus/downsyndrome.html. Accessed June 2004.

4 Traumatically Disabled Children

▶▶▶ case presentation

Joe is a 5-year-old boy who sustained a serious traumatic brain injury 3 months ago when he was an unbelted, front-seat passenger in a motor vehicle crash. One week ago he was discharged from a rehabilitation facility to home. He depends on a gastrostomy tube for all of his hydration and nutrition. Upon discovering that his gastrostomy tube is out, his mother panics and calls 9-1-1. When EMS arrives, the EMT notes that Joe is in bed. He appears to be in a vegetative state, and his extremities are hypertonic and contracted.

  1. What should be the first intervention?

  2. What are some of the concerns about this patient who is entirely dependent on his feeding tube?

▼ case progression

Joe's airway, breathing, and circulation appear intact. His heart rate is 75 beats/min, respiration rate is 20 beats/min, and blood pressure is 120/80 mm Hg. Joe is transported to the emergency department to have his gastrostomy tube replaced.

    A wide range of disabilities are seen in traumatically disabled children. A child or adolescent can sustain a traumatic brain injury and/or a spinal cord injury. This adolescent sustained a severe traumatic brain injury. He is entirely dependent on his feeding tube for hydration and nutrition, and therefore reinsertion of his feeding tube is a priority. Some children may depend on their feeding tube for medications as well. Parents of special needs children are typically expert in the care of their child. However, some parents will call EMS when under stress, such as when a child has been home for only a short time, or when the parents are unable to transport their child to the hospital.

Traumatically Disabled Children

Unintentional injury is a leading cause of morbidity and mortality in children and adolescents. Each year, nearly 6,700 children are killed and more than 50,000 are permanently disabled by preventable injuries. In the past, trauma care for acutely ill children has focused primarily on emergency medical and surgical issues. Currently, the approach to care has broadened to include rehabilitation, which, if introduced early in the management of the injury, may decrease the associated morbidity. Following a major traumatic incident such as a severe head or spinal cord injury, short-term and long-term disabilities may result. Children with significant head or spinal cord injuries are usually discharged home following a period of time in a rehabilitation hospital. The rehabilitative regime at home may include physical, occupational, and/or speech therapy. Special equipment needs for these children may include orthopedic devices such as splints, mobilization devices such as wheelchairs, oxygen, mechanical ventilators, suction, a gastrostomy feeding tube and pump, a central intravenous catheter to deliver IV nutrition, or a ventricular peritoneal shunt (VP shunt) to prevent increased intracranial pressure.[1,2]

Potential medical problems include:
- Neurologic deterioration
- Feeding tube dislodgement
- Shunt failure
- Bowel obstruction
- Tracheostomy tube dislodgement
- Tracheal occlusion
- Central line malfunction
- Increased intracranial pressure
- Respiratory distress
- Pneumonia or sepsis

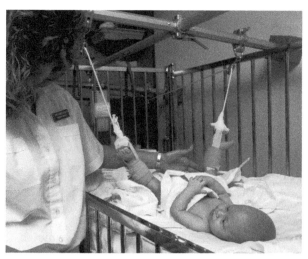

Figure 4-1 Some children with spinal cord lesions may wear special braces in the lower extremities.

Signs and Symptoms

- Signs and symptoms vary depending on the chronic condition created from the traumatic event and the equipment needed for survival
- Paraplegic and quadriplegic children have difficulty regulating their body temperature
- Wheelchair-bound children may be unaware of injuries and can sustain pressure sores
- Quadriplegics may have tracheostomies and be ventilator-dependent. They can suffer from the same respiratory conditions as any other child dependent on a ventilator: infection, obstructed tracheostomy tube, and equipment failure.

Home/Medical Management

- Wheelchairs
- IV or feeding pumps
- Supplemental oxygen
- Apnea monitors and/or suction
- Orthopedic/support devices
- Feeding catheters
- Pulse oximetry
- Ventilators

Treatment

Treatment depends on the type and severity of the lesion. The higher the spinal cord lesion, the more likely that the child needs a tracheostomy and mechanical ventilation. Also, these children are fed

through feeding tubes. Many children with spinal cord lesions will be in wheelchairs. Some of these children may wear special braces in the lower extremities (**Figure 4-1**). Children with traumatic brain injuries either will be mobile or, if in a persistent vegetative state, will be bed-bound. Most of these children will be receiving ongoing physical and occupational therapy to help with mobility and to learn activities of daily living. Some brain-injured children may have seizure disorders and will therefore be on antiseizure medications.

Prehospital Management

BLS Interventions
- Assessment and management of the ABCs
- Suction the oral airway or tracheostomy tube as necessary
- Assist the caregiver with changing the tracheostomy tube as necessary
- Provide supplemental oxygen as indicated (manual resuscitation if necessary)
- Provide humidified sterile normal saline if the patient has a tracheostomy tube

ALS Interventions
- Establish an IV or access central line if indicated
- Treat seizures per local EMS protocols
- Monitor cardiac status
- Decompress stomach by venting (opening) feeding tube if abdomen is distended
- Normal saline 20 cc/kg IV fluid bolus if hypoperfused

Caring for Children With . . .

Spinal Cord Injuries and/or Traumatic Brain Injury

1. Use caution when working with a child with known paralysis. In the event of trauma, carefully examine extremities for potential injuries, since the child will not be able to feel pain in paralyzed limbs. Also, tell the child which areas of the body are being assessed so as to not frighten him or her. Do not allow extremities to "dangle" or become "caught" during transfer of the child to the stretcher.

2. The flashing strobe lights on an ambulance can potentially trigger seizure activity in a child with a known seizure disorder. To avoid this, cover the child's eyes or turn off the response lights, if safety allows, when moving the child in and out of the emergency vehicle.

3. When moving a child with muscle contractures, do not attempt to "straighten" contracted extremities. Instead, support the child's body and extremities with pillows, towels, etc., in a position most comfortable for the patient.

4. Children with muscle contractures may have spasmodic muscle contractions (similar to the rapid jerking movement seen during seizure activity) when they are moved. This is an indication that the child is either frightened or experiencing pain. This reaction may be avoided by slowly, securely, and gently moving these children.

References

1. Batshaw M. *Your Child has a Disability*. Baltimore, MD: Paul H. Brookes Publishing; 1991.
2. Batshaw ML. *Children with Disabilities*, 5th ed. Baltimore, MD: Paul H. Brookes Publishing; 2002.

Resources

Brain Injury Association of America. Available at: http://www.biausa.org/Pages/home.html. Accessed June 2004.

CDC—Traumatic Brain Injury. Available at: http://www.cdc.gov/ncipc/factsheets/tbi.htm. Accessed June 2004.

NINDS Traumatic Brain Injury Information Page. Available at:
http://www.ninds.nih.gov/health_and_medical/disorders/tbi_doc.htm. Accessed June 2004.

The Rehabilitation Research Center for Traumatic Brain Injury and Spinal Cord Injury. Available at:
http://www.tbi-sci.org/main.html. Accessed June 2004.

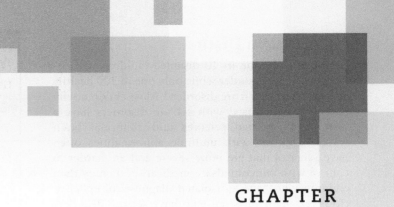

Neurologic Diseases in Children

5

Paul is a 10-year-old boy with hydrocephalus and a ventriculoperitoneal (VP) shunt since birth. He is a formally premature infant born at 25 weeks gestational age. He sustained a bleed in his head at birth and had a shunt placed to decrease intracranial pressure. He is developmentally delayed and has mild cerebral palsy. Paul began seizing that morning and his caregiver administered rectal Valium, but Paul continued to seize. His caregiver called 9-1-1. Upon arrival, the paramedic notes a child in bed having tonic-clonic motor activity. The child's caregiver states that he has been seizing for at least 30 minutes.

1. What should be the prehospital provider's primary concern?
2. What are the likely precipitators of this child's seizure?
3. What precautions should EMS take during the transport?

▼ case progression

The primary concern in this seizing child is his airway and breathing. The child's respiratory rate is 8 breaths/min, his heart rate is 120 beats/min, and his blood pressure is 100/70 mm Hg. The paramedic puts the child on a monitor while his partner begins to bag-mask ventilate the boy. Maintaining the airway in a seizing child may be challenging because the soft tissues of the tongue and palate may occlude the airway. Also, a child who has been seizing for a long period of time and who may have been given a lot of antiepileptic medication may have a decreased respiratory effort. It is evident that this child's airway and breathing are compromised. His initial pulse oximetry reading is 82% in room air. The paramedics are so concerned about this child's airway and breathing that they prepare to intubate his trachea and to transport him to the hospital. Transport precautions that should be taken in a child with cerebral palsy include securing the child to the stretcher in a position of comfort and avoiding forcing his extremities to lay straight. Padding is important for comfort and to prevent injury. Also, consideration should be given to turning off the flashing lights as there is some evidence that they may induce seizures in some children.

    <u>Neurologic diseases</u> in children include conditions such as seizure disorders, hydrocephalus, spina bifida, mental retardation, and developmental delays, among others. Other defects, such as cerebral palsy, are centered in the brain and result from a lack of oxygen to this vital organ before it has fully matured (approximately 16 years of age). The origin of a specific neuromuscular disease can vary from damage to the spinal cord, to peripheral nerves, to the neuromuscular junction, or to the muscle itself. The damage can be congenital or acquired.

▪▪ Seizure Disorders

Approximately one in 10 disabled children will develop a seizure disorder while only one in 200 healthy children have a seizure disorder.1 Most children who have been diagnosed with seizure disorders have a history of repeated seizures and abnormal brain waves. Children with multiple abnormalities often have seizures that are more severe and are harder to control with anticonvulsant medication therapy than children who have an isolated diagnosis of epilepsy. However, many children who have seizure disorders do have normal intelligence, and their seizures are well controlled by anticonvulsant medications.2 There are two categories of seizure disorders: generalized seizures and partial seizures (Table 5-1).

Generalized Seizures

Tonic-clonic seizures or grand mal are the most common type. The child may experience an aura prior to the beginning of a seizure. Initially the child's muscles become rigid then progress to rhythmic jerking. During this activity, the child is unconscious. The seizure can last from 30 seconds to 5 minutes or longer. Complete muscle relaxation following the seizure may result in incontinence. Finally, the child will be in a postictal state where he or she is lethargic or asleep.

Absence seizures or petite mal are less common. This type of seizure usually occurs later in childhood or adolescence. There are no focal tonic-clonic movements. Seizure presentation usually includes a normally behaving child with sudden halt in activity, a vacant look, and lack of awareness. This type of seizure activity may occur 100 times per day.[1]

Myoclonic seizures are characterized by sudden startle-like episodes in which the body flexes or briefly extends. The most common type of myoclonic seizure is known as infantile spasms. Onset is typically 3 to 6 months of age. Myoclonic seizures often occur in clusters of 8 to 10, multiple times a day. These seizures are difficult to control and are associated with a poor prognosis.[1]

Partial Seizures

Partial seizure activity is limited to one part of the brain. The presentation of the seizing child depends on the location of the abnormal electrical activity in the brain.

Simple partial seizures occur when the child is conscious and aware while experiencing episodes of partial seizures. Complex partial seizures are associated with a loss of consciousness. Psychomotor seizures are the most common type of partial seizure activity. The child usually first experiences hallucinations involving an unusual taste, smell, or sound. Feelings of anger or fear are experienced following the seizure, although it is uncommon to see acting out of these feelings. The actual seizure activity presents

Table 5-1 Seizure Summary	
Type of Seizure	**Features**
Generalized seizures	
Tonic-clonic (grand mal)	Aura, muscle rigidity, rhythmic jerking, postictal state
	Lasts anywhere from 30 seconds to 5 minutes or longer
Absence (petit mal)	Vacant look and is unaware of anything, returns to normal
	No focal tonic-clonic movements
Myoclonic	Sudden startle-like episodes (body briefly flexes or extends)
	Occurs in clusters of 8–10, often multiple times a day
Partial Seizures	
Simple partial seizures	Limited to one part of brain, affected area directly related to muscle group involved
	Child is aware
Complex partial seizures	Similar to simple, except that the child is unconscious
Psychomotor seizure	Hallucinations involving an unusual taste, smell, or sound. Feelings of fear or anger.
	Repetitive fine-motor actions such as lip smacking or eye blinking
	May progress to tonic-clonic seizure

with repetitive fine-motor actions such as lip smacking, eye blinking, or mumbling. The length of the seizure usually lasts a few minutes; however, it may progress to a tonic-clonic seizure.

Signs and Symptoms

- May be unresponsive
- Motor movements of extremities
- Staring spells (in certain types of nonmotor seizures)
- Eye deviation
- Compromised airway

(See Table 5-1 for specific signs of different types of seizures.)

Treatment

Treatment of children with seizure disorders most often involves the use of antiepileptic medications. A very small number of children have vagal nerve stimulators, an implantable device that is "turned on" with a magnet. A small number of children with severe seizure disorders are on a ketogenic diet. This diet has been shown to decrease the frequency of seizures, but is a very difficult diet to maintain, so it is only used for children whose seizures cannot be controlled by medication.

Home/Medical Management

- Antiepileptic medications (e.g., rectal Valium)

Prehospital Management

BLS Interventions
- Assessment and management of airway, breathing, and circulation
- Oxygen
- Position of comfort
- Assist parent or caregiver in the administration of home rectal Valium if not already given
- Transport to home hospital if local protocols allow

ALS Interventions
- Assessment and management of airway, breathing, and circulation
- If in respiratory failure, consider endotracheal intubation
- Intravenous access
- Intravenous fluid and/or antiepileptic medication as per local EMS protocol or medical control

Hydrocephalus

Hydrocephalus is an excessive build-up of cerebrospinal fluid (CSF) within the part of the brain known as ventricles (**Figure 5-1**). This excess CSF results in an abnormal dilatation of the ventricles and harmful pressure on the brain tissue. In 2000, the rate of hydrocephalus was 2.4/10,000 live births.[3] Hydrocephalus can be congenital or acquired. Congenital hydrocephalus is often associated with the neural tube defect, spina bifida (Myelomeningocele). Acquired hydrocephalus can result from trauma, infections (such as meningitis), intraventricular hemorrhage, brain tumor, or scar tissue formation.

Management of a child with hydrocephalus typically includes placement of a CSF shunt in order to drain off excessive CSF from the brain. This prevents increased intracranial pressure and possibly death. The shunt is surgically placed in the ventricle and threaded to the right atrium of the heart, or more

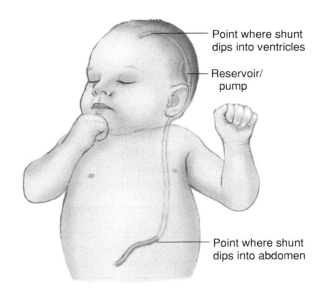

Figure 5-1 Hydrocephalus.

commonly to the peritoneal cavity, and is known as a ventriculoperitoneal (VP) shunt. Potential major complications that can occur in children with CSF shunts include obstruction, infection, or overdrainage. Obstruction, or plugging of the shunt, can occur at any point within the system. Shunt obstruction can be caused by blood clots, brain fragment, or tumor cells. Obstruction of the peritoneal end can be caused by loops of bowel, scar tissue, or other structures. Other complications can include shunt separation, growth of the child resulting in inlet or outlet changes, and shunt infection.

A second shunt complication is infection. Shunt infections typically occur within 1 to 2 months of surgical placement or revision. In this case, the child may present with a fever and possibly unusual redness or swelling along the shunt system. If left untreated, the condition may develop into sepsis, encephalitis, peritonitis, or meningitis.

Finally, overdrainage of CSF can result in the child experiencing a headache that worsens on standing and is relieved upon lying down. In addition, the child may present with symptoms of nausea, vomiting, drowsiness, and vision changes.

Signs and Symptoms

- Headache
- Nausea
- Vomiting
- Fever
- Blurred vision
- Irritability
- Loss of coordination
- Decreased level of consciousness

Treatment

Treatment depends on the cause of the malfunction. Shunt failure either by obstruction or malfunction can lead to increased intracranial pressure (ICP). Elevation of ICP is treated with medications, mild hyperventilation (to achieve a $PaCO_2$ of 35 on an arterial blood gas), and neurosurgical procedures to drain the fluid. The definitive treatment is surgery. When the shunt is obstructed, it is replaced or reconstructed surgically. If a shunt is infected, then it is replaced and the child is put on antibiotics intravenously.

Home/Medical Management

- There is no home equipment or medications for these children as the VP shunt is internal.

Prehospital Management

BLS Interventions
- Assessment and management of airway, breathing, and circulation
- Oxygen
- Position of comfort
- Transport to home hospital if local protocols allow it

ALS Interventions
- Assessment and management of airway, breathing, and circulation
- If in respiratory failure, consider endotracheal intubation
- Intravenous access
- Intravenous fluid and/or antiepileptic medication if patient is seizing as per local EMS protocol or medical control

Spina Bifida

Spina bifida refers to a gap in the vertebral arches (**Figure 5-2**). There are two basic types: spina bifida occulta, the more common but milder form, and spina bifida associated with malformation of the spine and attachment of a sac, a condition known as myelomeningocele. Since the recommendation that all women of child-bearing age take folic acid and certain foods were enriched with folic acid, the incidence of spina bifida in the United States has declined. The rate of spina bifida in the United States was approximately 2.1/10,000 live births in year 2000.[3]

This defect occurs around the third week of fetal development in utero. Clinical presentation depends on the level of the defect. Spina bifida often results in partial or complete paralysis and loss of sensory function, though this is not always symmetrical with motor loss. In addition, the child may present with loss of

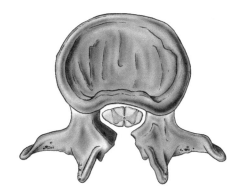

Figure 5-2 Spina bifida.

bladder or bowel control, cognitive impairments, visual deficits, and seizure disorders. Bladder and bowel dysfunction is very common among children with spina bifida. In such cases, there is incomplete emptying of the bladder, predisposing the child to urinary tract infections. Management of such cases requires emptying of the bladder by urinary catheterization, several times a day. Hydrocephalus associated with Arnold-Chiari malformation (displacement of the brain stem and part of cerebellum downward through the foramen magnum) occurs in greater than two thirds of children with spina bifida.[4]

Research has shown that children and adults with spina bifida have a greater risk of potentially developing an allergy to latex.[5-8] The reason for this is not certain, but multiple exposures to latex through the many medical procedures they require is often cited. Therefore, every child with spina bifida should be treated with latex-free equipment.

Signs and Symptoms

Signs and symptoms of spina bifida depend on the spinal level of the lesion and associated anomalies. These can include:
- Paralysis
- Decreased and lack of sensation below the level of the spinal lesion
- Seizures
- Urinary incontinence

Home/Medical Management

- Wheelchairs
- Colostomy or ileostomy
- Multiple medications
- Splints for contractions
- Urinary catheters
- CSF shunt

Treatment

Children with spina bifida can suffer from complications from their condition. This includes urinary tract infections (UTI), bowel obstruction, and CSF shunt failure or infection. People with spina bifida are susceptible to UTIs because they catheterize themselves frequently. UTIs are treated with antibiotics. Bowel obstruction occurs most often in people with previous bowel surgeries and is relieved surgically. Shunt failure is treated surgically as well.

Prehospital Management

- Use latex-free equipment for BLS and ALS interventions.

BLS Interventions
- Assessment and management of airway, breathing, and circulation
- Oxygen
- Position of comfort
- Transport to home hospital if local protocols allow

ALS Interventions
- Assessment and management of airway, breathing, and circulation
- If in respiratory failure, consider endotracheal intubation
- Intravenous access
- Intravenous fluid and/or antiepileptic medication if patient is seizing as per local EMS protocol or medical control

Mental Retardation

Mental retardation is a disability characterized by significant limitations both in intellectual functioning and in adaptive behavior as expressed in conceptual, social, and practical adaptive skills. This disability originates before the age of 18.[9] An estimated 1% to 3% of the population is affected.[10] Mental retardation develops as a result of prenatal problems, or injury or disease that occurs during the developmental years. Down syndrome is the most common cause of mental retardation.[11] This is a developmentally nonprogressive disorder that impairs the child's ability to adapt to his or her surroundings. The primary goal of treatment is to develop the child's potential to the fullest through special education and training.

Developmental Delay

Developmental delay is failure to achieve age-appropriate milestones with atypical neurodevelopment impairment. A child who is developmentally delayed usually has suffered from a prolonged illness or was born prematurely. These children have the potential to "catch up" and to eventually progress normally with their growth and development.

Signs and Symptoms

- Cognitive ability lower than expected for age
- These children may become agitated more easily with strangers and strange situations

Home/Medical Management

Isolated mental retardation or developmental delay is typically an educational issue as opposed to a medical issue. These children are often in special education programs. Some of these children may have associated medical issues such as cerebral palsy, seizure disorders, or other congenital or genetic conditions (see specific medical disorders for treatment).

Prehospital Management

ALS and BLS Interventions
- Ask caregivers about the child's developmental level
- Treat the child as you would any child at that same level
- Seriously consider transporting the caregiver with the child

Cerebral Palsy (CP)

Cerebral palsy (CP) refers to a group of chronic nonprogressive disorders that are caused by damage to the motor centers of the brain in the early stages of life (Figure 5-3). Cerebral refers to the brain's two halves, or hemispheres, and palsy describes any disorder that impairs control of body movement. Damage or abnormal development to motor areas in the brain disables the brain's ability to adequately control movement and posture. A child with cerebral palsy has abnormal muscle tone and postures that can present as either muscular spasms or a lack of muscle tone. Other associated conditions include mental retardation, occurring in 50% to 60%, and seizure disorder, which affects 30% to 50% of this population.[12,13]

The prevalence of this condition ranges from 1.4 to 2.5/1,000 and has remained constant for many years.[14,15] It is estimated that more than 500,000 Americans have cerebral palsy.[16] Depending on the cause, cerebral palsy can be categorized as acquired cerebral palsy or congenital cerebral palsy.

Acquired cerebral palsy occurs in 10% to 20% of the children with CP and results from brain damage in the first few months or years of life. Causes include brain infections, such as meningitis or encephalitis, or trauma from a head injury. Congenital cerebral palsy accounts for the majority of cases of CP.[18] Causes include infections during pregnancy, severe jaundice in infants, Rh incompatibility, severe oxygen shortage

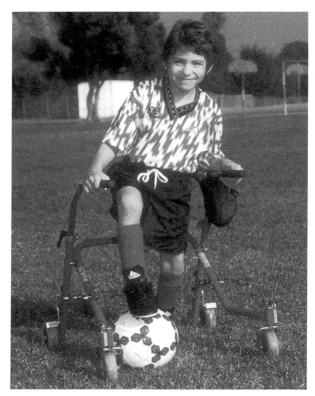

Figure 5-3 Cerebral palsy.

in the brain or trauma to the head during labor and delivery, or stroke.

Cerebral palsy is categorized according to impairment of the motor group into different types as follows. Spastic cerebral palsy is the most common type affecting 70% to 80% of patients with CP.[13] The condition is further classified, depending on the involvement of different group of muscles, as spastic hemiplegia, diplegia, and quadriplegia. Characteristics of spastic CP include muscles that are stiff and permanently contracted. These children may also experience uncontrollable shaking of their extremities.

Dyskinetic or athetoid cerebral palsy accounts for 10% to 15% of the cases.[13] The condition affects the whole body and presents with uncontrolled, slow movements. A characteristic feature of this condition is involuntary movements. A subtype of dyskinetic is athetoid CP, which presents with rapid jerky movements and writhing slow movements. It is classically associated with bilirubin encephalopathy.[19] Ataxic cerebral palsy is a relatively rare form affecting the sense of balance and depth perception. There is no cure for cerebral palsy. Instead, management is focused on improving the child's capabilities and quality

of life. Medications are available to control seizure activity and muscle spasms.

Orthopedic devices and surgery can improve or help to control muscle balance and contractures. In addition, various treatment modalities such as speech, occupational, physical, and behavioral therapies can enhance the child's abilities to accomplish activities of daily living.

There are several long-term complications relating to cerebral palsy. Incontinence, the most common complication, is caused by poor control over the muscles that keep the bladder closed. Poor control of the throat, mouth, and tongue can sometimes lead to drooling and increases the risk for aspiration. Medications to reduce the flow of saliva are available. Difficulty with eating and swallowing can cause poor nutrition. In severe cases, an artificial feeding tube may need to be placed in order to provide nutrients to the child.

Signs and Symptoms

- Signs and symptoms of cerebral palsy vary with the type and severity of the disorder.
- Signs and symptoms depend on whether the child is dependent on equipment for survival.

Treatment

Children with cerebral palsy can suffer from a variety of problems. Home treatment depends on the severity of the condition and the associated conditions. Some of these problems include respiratory infections, aspiration, feeding tube dislodgement, and seizures. Many of these children are in wheelchairs and need assistance with their activities of daily living. Some are on medications to control their contractures and to control seizures. Some are also fed by feeding tubes.

Home/Medical Management

- Wheelchairs
- Colostomy or ileostomy
- Multiple medications
- Feeding catheters
- Splints for contractures
- Feeding pump
- Suction
- CSF shunt
- Intrathecal baclofen pump

BLS Interventions

- Assessment and management of the airway, breathing, and circulation
- Suction the oral airway or tracheostomy tube as necessary
- Provide supplemental oxygen or manual ventilations as indicated
- Place the actively seizing child in a lateral position to prevent aspiration
- Provide a safe environment for an actively seizing child
- Observe for signs and symptoms of CSF shunt failure; if possible, transport child sitting up to decrease intracranial pressure
- Realize that fever can be an indication of a CSF infection or urinary tract infection

- Assist the child's caregiver with decompressing the stomach by venting (opening) the feeding tube if the abdomen is distended
- Assist the caregiver with discontinuing any supplemental NG or GT feedings (clamp off feeding catheter), transport child sitting up to prevent aspiration

ALS Interventions

- Intubate the child's trachea if necessary
- Establish IV access or access a central line if indicated (if local EMS protocols allow)
- Treat seizures per local protocol
- Administer Valium 0.05 to 0.1 mg/kg IV while monitoring cardiac status as arrhythmias may be present in CSF shunt failure

Neurologic Disorders

1. If a child has diagnosed epilepsy, the parents may have already given a rectal suppository of an anticonvulsant medication to stop seizure activity prior to EMS arrival. These medications may include Ativan, Valium, or Diastat. In this case, monitor the child for potential respiratory depression and contact medical control prior to giving additional anticonvulsant medication.

2. Always assume any child with spina bifida has a latex allergy or sensitivity. Use latex-free products while caring for these patients. Items in your ambulance that may contain latex include gloves, blood pressure cuffs, stethoscopes, cervical collars, IV tubing, oxygen tubing, etc. Read the labels on your supplies to determine if any of these items contain latex. Reactions can range from localized redness to anaphylaxis.

3. When moving a child with muscle contractures, do not attempt to "straighten" contracted extremities. Instead, support the child's body and extremities with pillows, towels, etc. in a position most comfortable for the patient.

4. Children with muscle contractures may have spasmodic muscle contractions (similar to the rapid jerking movement seen during seizure activity) when they are moved. This is an indication that the child is either frightened or experiencing pain. This reaction may be avoided by slowly, securely, and gently moving these children.

5. Be careful to support the airway of children who normally have difficulty handling oral secretions (e.g., severe cases of cerebral palsy, mental retardation).

6. The flashing strobe lights on an ambulance can potentially trigger seizure activity in a child with a known seizure disorder. To avoid this, cover the child's eyes or turn off the response lights, if safety allows, when moving the child in and out of the emergency vehicle.

7. Use caution working with a child with known paralysis. In the event of a trauma, carefully examine extremities for potential injuries since the child will not be able to feel pain in the paralyzed areas. Also, verbalize to the child which areas of the body are being assessed so as to not frighten him or her. Do not allow extremities to "dangle" or become "caught" during transfer of the child.

References

1. Batshaw M. *Your Child Has a Disability.* Baltimore, MD: Paul H. Brookes Publishing; 1991:92.
2. Brown L. Seizure disorders, In: Batshaw M. *Children with Disabilities,* 4th ed. Baltimore, MD: Paul H. Brookes Publishing; 1997:553–593.
3. Nation Vital Statistics Report. Births: Final Draft for 2002. Table 49, vol. 50, no. 5, Feb. 12. Available at: http://www.cdc.gov/nchs/data/nvsr/nvsr50/nvsr 50_05.pdf. Accessed June 2004.
4. Griebel ML, Oakes WJ, Worley G. The Chiari malformation associated with meningomyelocele. In: Rekate HL, ed. *Comprehensive Management of Spina Bifida.* Boca Raton, FL: CRC Press; 1991:67–92.
5. Banta JV, Bonanni C, Prebluda J. Latex anaphylaxis during spinal surgery in children with myelomeningocele. *Dev Med Child Neurol* 1993; 35:543–548.
6. Kelly KJ, Pearson ML, Kurup VP, Havens PL, Byrd RS, Setlock MA, Butler JC, Slater JE, Grammer LC, Resneck A, et al. A cluster of anaphylactic reactions in children with spina bifida during general anesthesia: epidemiologic features, risk factors and latex hypersensitivity. *J Allergy Clin Immunol* 1994; 94:53–61.
7. Ellsworth PI, Merguerian PA, Klein RB, Rozycki AA. Evaluation and risk factors of latex allergy in spina bifida patients: is it preventable? *J Urol* 1993; 150:691–693.
8. Nieto A, Estornell F, Mazon A, Reig C, Nieto A, Garcia-Ibarra F. Allergy to latex in spina bifida: a multivariate study of associated factors in 100 consecutive patients. *J Allergy Clin Immunol* 1996; 98:501–507.
9. American Association of Mental Retardation. Definition of Mental Retardation, 2002. Available at: www.aamr.org/Policies/faq_mental_retardation.shtml. Accessed June 2004.
10. Heath Central. General Health Encyclopedia, Mental retardation 1998. Available at: www.healthcentral.com/mhc/top/001523.cfm. Accessed June 2004.
11. Batshaw ML, Shapiro BK. Mental retardation. In: Batshaw M, ed. *Children with Disabilities,* 4th ed. Baltimore, MD: Paul H. Brookes Publishing; 1997:335–360.
12. Eicher PS, Batshaw ML. Cerebral palsy. *Pediatr Clin N Am* 1993; 40:537–549.
13. Taft LT. Cerebral palsy. *Pediatr Rev* 1995; 16:411–418.
14. Cummins SK, Nelson KB, Grether JK, Velie EM. Cerebral palsy in four northern California counties, births 1983–1985. *J Pediatr* 1993; 123:230–237.
15. Hagberg B, Hagberg G, Olow I. The changing panorama of cerebral palsy in Sweden: VI. Prevalence and origin during the birth year period 1983–1986. *Acta Paediatr* 1993; 82:387–393.
16. National Information Center for Children and Youth with Disabilities, Cerebral palsy, Factsheet 2, 1994. Available at: www.nichcy.org/pubs/factshe/fs2txt.htm. Accessed June 2004.
17. Scher MS, Belfar H, Martin J, Painter MJ. Destructive brain lesions of presumed fetal onset: Antepartum causes of cerebral palsy. *Pediatrics* 1991; 88:898–906.
18. MacDonald MG. Hidden risks: Early discharge and bilirubin toxicity due to G6PD deficiency. *Pediatrics* 1995; 8:20–24.

Resources

Batshaw M. *Children with Disabilities,* 5th ed. Baltimore, MD: Paul H. Brookes Publishing; 2003.
Epilepsy Foundation. Available at: www.efa.org. Accessed February 2004.
American Epilepsy Society. Available at: http://www.aesnet.org. Accessed February 2004.
United Cerebral Palsy. Available at: http://www.ucp.org. Accessed February 2004.

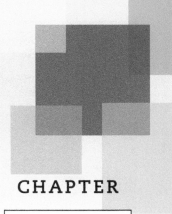

CHAPTER

6

Hematology and Oncology Diseases in Children

▶▶▶ case presentation

Steve is a 2-year-old boy with a history of sickle cell disease. His mother brought him to the pediatrician's office because he had a fever of 102°F at home. While in the pediatrician's waiting area, he becomes limp. The pediatrician calls 9-1-1 when she notes that Steve is pale and difficult to arouse. When the prehospital responders arrive, they too note a pale and listless child. They immediately place him on a monitor and note that his heart rate is 200 beats/min, his respiratory rate is 40 breaths/min, and his blood pressure is 90/50 mm Hg. The paramedics are unable to obtain a pulse oximetry reading.

1. What are the most important prehospital interventions?
2. What is the most likely diagnosis in this child?

▼ case progression

Prior to transport, the prehospital responders administer oxygen and place an IV. They begin an infusion of 20 cc/kg of normal saline. They prepare to transport the child for transport to his home hospital. Any child with sickle cell disease and a fever should be considered at high risk of serious bacterial infection. The most likely diagnosis in this child with sickle cell disease with fever and ill appearance is sepsis. Therefore, once this child has been stabilized at the scene, this child should be immediately transported and antibiotic therapy initiated. Children with sickle cell disease are at high risk for infection with encapsulated bacteria such as *Streptococcus pneumoniae* and *Haemophilus influenza*. Fortunately, many children with sickle cell disease are immunized against these organisms, but even still can become infected. Left untreated, these children can die within a matter of hours. Therefore, fever in these children is always considered an emergency.

Sickle Cell Disease

Sickle cell anemia (SCA) is an inherited, chronic, severe disease resulting from a disorder of the red blood cells (Figure 6-1). SCA predominantly affects the African-American population with a prevalence of about 1 in 375 individuals.[1] One in 10 African Americans carry the trait. Abnormal hemoglobin S (HgbS) replaces all or part of the normal hemoglobin, which causes a change in the oxygen-carrying hemoglobin inside red blood cells; these cells become distorted, forming a rigid "banana" or "sickle" shape that can clog blood vessels. Because sickle cells cannot slide through vessels as normal cells do, it results in clumping, thrombosis, arterial obstruction, increased blood

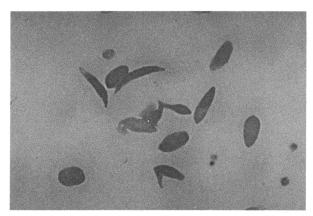

Figure 6-1 Sickle cell anemia.

viscosity, hemolysis, and eventually tissue ischemia and necrosis. Mild hypoxia, dehydration, cold, extreme fatigue, infection, fever, or strenuous exercise can cause the red blood cells to change from round to crescent shaped.

There are several types of "crises" in a child with sickle cell disease. One of the most common is the vaso-occlusive or pain crisis, which results when sickled cells occlude blood vessels, most often capillaries, thus decreasing the circulation of oxygenated blood and producing infarcts of adjacent tissue. This is often referred to as a painful episode, event, or crisis. These sickled cells also may become trapped within the vessels in the brain (causing a stroke), in the cardiac circulation (causing a myocardial infarction), or in the lungs (causing a chest crisis).

Another type of crisis only seen in young children is splenic sequestration crisis. This occurs when there is a sudden enlargement of the spleen caused by trapped sickled red blood cells. The result is a sequestration (pooling) of a large blood volume in the spleen potentially leading to shock and death. This problem typically occurs in children less than 6 years of age because by that time, a child with sickle cell disease (SCD) has an infarcted spleen that is no longer functional. Aplastic crisis occurs when the bone marrow slows or stops new red blood cell production. This can dramatically and dangerously drop the hemoglobin level.

Sepsis is caused by a combination of impaired immunologic functions, most notably an early loss of normal splenic function. The spleen functions to filter out encapsulated bacteria that may be circulating in the bloodstream. If the spleen is not functioning properly, these bacteria are then free to cause infection and sepsis, and this contributes to a markedly increased frequency of blood infection in patients with sickle cell disease. A young child with SCA presenting with a fever must be evaluated immediately by a physician and started on aggressive antibiotic therapy. Consider this child to have a medically emergent condition.

Signs and Symptoms

- Pain
- Fever
- Abdominal pain
- Pallor
- Shortness of breath, cough, or fever if in chest crisis

Treatment

Young children with sickle cell disease are often on prophylactic antibiotics (penicillin) and folic acid. They require frequent visits to their hematologists to monitor their illness. Those children who have had a stroke may have a central venous catheter so that they can receive monthly blood transfusions to keep their ratio of sickled cells below a certain percentage to prevent subsequent strokes. Recently, bone marrow transplant has been used as a therapy for a few children with some success.

Home/Medical Management

- Some children are on prophylactic doses of penicillin
- Some children are on folic acid
- Some children are on other medications such as urea
- Children on transfusion protocols may have central venous lines

Prehospital Management

BLS Interventions
- Assessment and management of airway, breathing, and circulation
- Provide supplemental oxygen
- Place in position of comfort
- Place warm compresses over swollen joints during a pain crisis

ALS Interventions
- Start an IV
- Give a 20 cc/kg normal saline fluid bolus if patient presents with signs of shock
- Consider analgesic medication, such as morphine 0.1 mg/kg IV, for pain crisis if local EMS protocols allow
- Consider other pain modalities as well, such as warm packs over the parts of the body affected by the vaso-oclusive crisis

Hemophilia

A person with hemophilia has a missing or low supply of one of the factors needed for normal blood clotting. It is estimated that more than 15,000 people in the

United States have hemophilia.[2,3] A surveillance study conducted in six states estimated the incidence of hemophilia A and B to be 1 in 5,032 live male births during the period of 1982 to 1991.[2] Hemophilia may be mild, moderate, or severe. About 60% of persons with hemophilia are of the severe type. These people are at risk for bleeding after trauma or injury and at times bleed spontaneously. About 15% of persons with hemophilia have the moderate type and 25% have the mild type. In these cases, excessive bleeding is still common but may go undetected until after a traumatic injury or surgery.

The hemophilia gene is carried by females on one of their X chromosomes, and if passed to their male offspring will cause the disease. In about one third of all cases there is no family history of the disease, and hemophilia occurs as the result of a new or spontaneous mutation. Any male who inherits the defective chromosome has hemophilia. This is because males, unlike females, have only one X chromosome.

Signs and Symptoms

- Bleeding at site of trauma
- Swollen joint if bleed is into a joint
- Signs and symptoms of head injury if bleed is in the brain
- If significant blood loss, will see signs of increased heart rate, increased respiratory rate and possibly low blood pressure

Treatment

Treatments for hemophilia patients include prophylactic administration of a clotting factor on a regular basis and administration of a clotting factor when active bleeding occurs. Genetically engineered recombinant factors do not use blood in their development. This is why recombinant clotting factors are the safest factor products available today. The risks of receiving clotting factors made from blood products include HIV infection (which is rare now since new viral screening and purification methods have made blood supplies safer) and hepatitis. It may be especially urgent to expedite the transport of these children to ensure optimal availability of the factor required to control bleeding. Potential problems in children with hemophilia for which parents call for emergency help include uncontrolled bleeding, head injury, caregivers unable to obtain vascular access, and adverse reaction to clotting factor.

Home/Medical Management

- Syringes for administering factor at home
- Vascular access equipment
- Central line (commonly implanted)
- Vials of clotting factor

Prehospital Management

BLS Interventions

- Assessment and management of airway, breathing, and circulation
- Administer oxygen if necessary
- Attempt to control bleeding (direct pressure, elevation, etc.)
- Gently handle the patient to avoid bruising
- Assist parent in administering factor if local EMS protocol allows it
- Transfer the child to his home hospital if possible

ALS Interventions

- Establish a peripheral IV or access the patient's central line if IV fluids and/or IV drug administration are necessary (follow local protocols)
- Administer a 20 cc/kg normal saline IV fluid bolus for signs and symptoms of shock
- Assist the family in the administration of the child's clotting factor
- Monitor the child for adverse reactions to the factor (allergic reaction, difficulty breathing, sudden fever)
- Consider transport to the home hospital if local EMS protocols allow

Leukemia

Leukemia is the most common form of childhood cancer. Other less common types of cancer in childhood include lymphoma, tumors of the nervous system and bone cancer as well as many other types of cancer.[4,5] In the United States between 1990 and 1998, leukemia represented 30% of all cancers among children under 15 years of age.[5] Each year the number of children in the U.S. diagnosed with leukemia is greater than 3,250.[5] However, because of early diagnosis and improved treatment regimens, the 5-year survival rate has increased to 77%.[6]

Leukemia is a malignant disease of the bone marrow and blood, which is characterized by the uncontrolled growth of white blood cells. Depending on the cell type involved, leukemia is categorized into four major groups as acute or chronic and myelogenous or lymphocytic leukemia. Among these, the most common form of leukemia in children under the age of 15 years is acute lymphocytic leukemia (ALL),[5] which is a rapidly progressing disease that results in the accumulation of immature, functionless white blood cells in the marrow and blood. The marrow often no longer produces enough normal red and white blood cells and platelets. Abnormal cells replace red blood cells, which results in anemia. Abnormal cells and/or poorly functioning cells also replace normal white blood cells. A dramatically low white blood cell (WBC) count impairs the body's ability to fight off bacterial, viral, or fungal infections. Platelet production severely slows, resulting in poor blood clotting and bruising. Chronic leukemia progresses more slowly and permits greater numbers of more mature, functional cells to be made.

Potential life-threatening problems in children with leukemia include infection, low platelet counts, and tumor in the cerebrospinal fluid. Because the immune systems of these children are severely impaired, they are susceptible to infection and sepsis. Fever in a child with a low WBC is considered an emergency and necessitates evaluation and treatment. As the WBC can be low, platelets can be dangerously low as well, and sometimes these children need platelet transfusions to prevent uncontrollable bleeding.

Signs and Symptoms

- Pallor
- Fever
- Listlessness
- Bone pain without apparent trauma
- Increased heart rate

Treatment

Treatment for leukemia and many other forms of cancer includes chemotherapy, radiation, and bone marrow transplant. Chemotherapy involves the use of powerful drugs in various combinations to kill abnormal cells and/or to slow their growth, thus giving normal cells a chance to grow and function. Radiation is often used in combination with chemotherapy depending on the treatment protocol. Bone marrow transplantation is a treatment for certain types of leukemias as well as relapsed leukemia and is an option provided a suitable donor is found, which can either be the patient or another person. This procedure involves the injection of healthy bone marrow into the patient's bloodstream, ultimately entering the bone. The goal is for healthy cells and platelets to begin developing.

Home/Medical Management

- Central lines
- IV or feeding pumps
- Feeding catheters
- Oral medications

Prehospital Management

BLS Interventions

- Assess and manage airway, breathing, and circulation
- Provide supplemental oxygen or assisted ventilations as appropriate
- Wear a mask to protect the patient from possible infections
- Gentle handling of the patient to avoid bruising
- For terminally ill children, determination of DNR status—follow local protocol

ALS Interventions

- Establish a peripheral IV or access the patient's central line if IV fluids and/or IV drug administration are necessary (follow local protocols)
- Administer a 20 cc/kg normal saline IV fluid bolus for signs and symptoms of shock
- Consider the use of inotropes if repeated normal saline fluid boluses do not improve circulation
- Give pain medication when appropriate, morphine 0.1 mg/kg IV if allowed by local EMS protocol

Caring for Children With . . .

Hematologic/Oncologic Diseases

Sickle cell disease

1. Recognize that a vaso-occlusive crisis is very painful. Contact medical control early to request medication for pain management.
2. Because of a poorly or nonfunctioning spleen, these children are very susceptible to infections. Consider fever to be a medical emergency that must be aggressively treated with antibiotics.
3. A young child complaining of severe abdominal pain may be having a splenic sequestration, which can be life-threatening.
4. IV access may be extremely challenging because these children frequently require IV therapy.
5. Any fever should be considered an emergency because the child's ability to fight an infection is impaired due to a poorly functioning or nonfunctioning spleen.

Hemophilia

1. It is in the child's best interest to be transported to his home hospital, as certain types of clotting factor are rare and the home hospital will usually have the type of clotting factor that the child requires.
2. It must be emphasized that bleeding will *not* stop with conventional methods. The missing clotting factor must be administered intravenously.
3. Some children have such a severe clotting factor deficiency that they are given a dose daily as a precaution. These children usually have implanted central lines.

Leukemia

1. Children will generally have a central line during their chemotherapy regime.
2. Consider fever a medical emergency. Chemotherapy can dramatically decrease the child's ability to fight off infection.
3. Providers should wear masks and gloves because the child's immune system is greatly compromised when undergoing chemotherapy treatments.

References

1. Bowman JE, Murray RF Jr. *Genetic variation and disorders in people of African origin.* Baltimore, MD: Johns Hopkins University Press; 1990:196–201.
2. Soucie JM, Evatt B, Jackson D. Occurrence of hemophilia in the United States. The Hemophilia Surveillance System Project Investigators. *Am J Hematol* 1998;59:288–294.
3. National Institute of Health, National Heart, Lung and Blood Institute. Hemophilia, May 13, 1996. Available at: http://www.nhlbi.nih.gov/health/ public/blood/other/hemophel.htm. Accessed June 2004.
4. Tata Memorial Center–Pediatric Center. Pediatric Cancer (table). Available at: *http://www.tatamemorialcentre.com/reg1.htm.* Accessed June 2004.
5. The Leukemia and Lymphoma Society. Disease information/Blood Related Cancers/About the Disease/Leukemia. Available at: www.leukemia-lymphoma.org. Accessed June 2004.
6. National Cancer Institute. Smith MA, Gloeckler-Ries LA, Gurney JG, Ross JA. SEER Pediatric Monograph. Leukemia. Available at: www.Seer.cancer.gov/publications/childhood/leukemia.pdf. Accessed June 2004.

Resources

National Hemophilia Foundation. Bleeding Disorders Information Center: Hemophilia. Available at: www.hemophilia.org. Accessed June 2004.

Sickle Cell Disease Association of America. Available at: http://www.sicklecelldisease.org. Accessed June 2004.

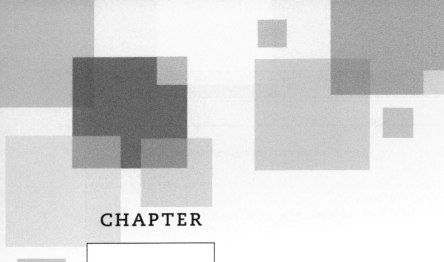

7 Immunologic Diseases in Children

▶▶▶ case presentation

Jay is a 13-year-old boy who has congenital HIV. He is living with an aunt. Jay told his aunt that he wasn't feeling well, so she takes his temperature and finds that he has a 103°F fever. He appears sick to her. She drives him to the hospital where he is immediately brought back to a room. His vital signs are temperature 102.7°F, heart rate 130 beats/min, respiratory rate of 30 breaths/min, blood pressure of 100/70 mm Hg, and a pulse oximetry reading of 91%. He is ill appearing.

1. What should be the emergency providers' first concern?
2. What is the most likely diagnosis?

▼ case progression

Blood cultures are drawn and IV antibiotics are administered. Because of his elevated respiratory rate and fever, Jay also gets a chest x-ray. He is found to have pneumonia. He is admitted to the hospital on IV antibiotics and oxygen.

■.■ HIV and AIDS

As of 2001 in the United States, 8,994 cases of AIDS, acquired immunodeficiency syndrome, have been reported among children 12 years of age and under.[1] In addition, 4,219 cases of AIDS were reported among young people from 13 to 19 years of age.[1] In 1999, AIDS ranked tenth among the leading causes of death for US children 5 to 9 years of age and seventh among young people 20 to 24 years of age.[2] Because the average period of time from human immunodeficiency virus (HIV) infection to the development of AIDS is 10 years, most young adults with AIDS were likely infected with HIV as adolescents.

AIDS is caused by HIV and is the most advanced stage of HIV infection. By killing or impairing cells of the immune system, HIV progressively destroys the body's ability to fight infections and certain cancers. Individuals diagnosed with AIDS are susceptible to life-threatening diseases called opportunistic infections. Effective January 1, 1993, the CDC revised its definition of AIDS to include all HIV-infected people who have fewer than 200 CD4+ T cells (healthy adults usually have CD4+ T-cell counts of 1,000 or more) or a CD4+ T-lymphocyte percentage of total lymphocytes of less than 14.[3] The definition in addition includes three clinical conditions—pulmonary tuberculosis, recurrent pneumonia, and invasive cervical cancer—and

23 existing clinical conditions in the AIDS surveillance case definition of 1987.[4] The most recent case definition for HIV infection revised in 2000 includes HIV nucleic acid (DNA or RNA) detection tests.[5] During the course of HIV infection, most people experience a gradual decline in the number of CD4+ T cells, although some individuals may have abrupt and dramatic drop in their CD4+ T-cell count. A person with a CD4+ T-cell count above 200 may experience some of the early symptoms of HIV disease. Others may have no symptoms even though their CD4+ T-cell count is below 200. Most AIDS-defining conditions are opportunistic infections, which rarely cause harm in healthy individuals. In people with AIDS, however, these infections are often severe and sometimes fatal because the immune system is too weak to fight off certain bacteria, viruses, and other microbes.

Opportunistic infections common in people with AIDS present with varied symptoms depending on the system involved. These include coughing, shortness of breath, fever, nausea, vomiting, abdominal cramps, difficult or painful swallowing, severe and persistent diarrhea, weight loss, extreme fatigue, and mental symptoms such as confusion and forgetfulness. Patient may also present with headaches, seizures, vision loss, lack of coordination, or coma. Although children with AIDS are susceptible to the same opportunistic infections as adults with the disease, they also experience severe forms of bacterial infections to which children are especially prone, such as conjunctivitis (pink eye), ear infections, and tonsillitis. People with AIDS are particularly prone to developing various cancers, especially those caused by viruses such as Kaposi's sarcoma and cervical cancer, or cancers of the immune system known as lymphomas. These cancers are usually more aggressive and difficult to treat in people with AIDS. Hallmarks of Kaposi's sarcoma in light-skinned people are circular brown, reddish, or purple spots that develop in the skin or in the mouth. In dark-skinned people, the spots are more pigmented.

HIV is spread most commonly by sexual contact with an infected partner. The virus can enter the body through the lining of the vagina, vulva, penis, rectum, or mouth during sex. Women can transmit HIV to their fetuses during pregnancy or birth. Approximately one quarter to one third of all untreated pregnant women infected with HIV will pass the infection to their babies. HIV also can be spread to babies through the breastmilk of mothers infected with the virus.

Signs and Symptoms

- Fever
- Shortness of breath
- Cough
- Dyspnea
- Pallor
- Abdominal pain
- Nausea/vomiting
- Headache
- Increased heart rate
- Increased respiratory rate

Treatment

Children with HIV infection are on antiviral medications. They are monitored by their physicians and their blood counts and viral loads followed. Many of these children live a long time with the disease and rarely require emergency medical attention. However, potential problems that would prompt families and caregivers to seek EMS transport include fever and/or sepsis, respiratory tract infections, GI bleeding, and dehydration.

Home/Medical Management

- Multiple medications
- Feeding catheter
- Central line IV or feeding pumps

Prehospital Management

BLS Interventions
- Assessment and management of airway, breathing, and circulation
- Provide supplemental oxygen as needed
- Recognize that any fever should be considered an emergency
- For DNR orders, follow local protocol and contact medical control for guidance

ALS Interventions
- Start an IV of normal saline, giving a 20 cc/kg fluid bolus for signs and symptoms of hypoperfusion (e.g., dehydration, sepsis)

EMS Tips
Caring for Children With . . .

Immunologic Diseases
1. Consider fever a medical emergency since these children's immune systems are greatly compromised. Sepsis can develop quickly.
2. The need for high-tech medical support may increase as the child's disease progresses.
3. It is not uncommon for IV access to be especially challenging in these children.

References

1. Center for Disease Control and Prevention. National Center for HIV, STD, and TB Prevention, Basic statistics, last revised February 2002. Available at: http://www.cdc.gov/hiv/stats.htm. Accessed June 2004.
2. Center for Disease Control and Prevention, National Center for Health Statistics, Leading causes of death, October, 2001/49(11), p. 14. Available at: http://www.cdc.gov/nchs/about/major/dvs/mortdata.htm. Accessed June 2005.
3. Center for Disease Control and Prevention. Revision of the CDC surveillance case definition for acquired immunodeficiency syndrome MMWR. 1987; 36:1S–15S.
4. Center for Disease Control and Prevention, MMWRs on HIV/AIDS and Classification/Case Definition, 1993 Revised Classification System for HIV Infection and Expanded Surveillance Case Definition for AIDS Among Adolescents and Adults. December 25, 1992; 41(51):961–962. Available at: http://www.cdc.gov/hiv/pubs/mmwr/classification.htm. Accessed June 2005.
5. Center for Disease Control and Prevention. Appendix: Revised Surveillance Case Definition for HIV Infection MMWR. Dec 10, 1999; 48(RR-13):29–31. Available at: http://www.cdc.gov/hiv/pubs/mmwr/classification.htm. Accessed June 2005.

Resources

CDC National Center for HIV, STD, and TB Prevention, Division of HIV/AIDs Prevention. Available at: http://www.cdc.gov/hiv/dhap.htm. Accessed June 2004.

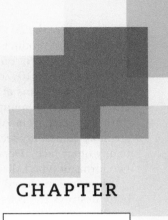

Endocrine Diseases in Children

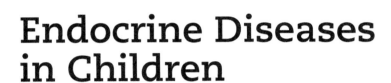

▶▶▶ case presentation

Paula is a 6-year-old girl with recently diagnosed insulin dependent diabetes mellitus (type 1 diabetes) who was found comatose by her mother. Panicked, Paula's mother calls 9-1-1. Upon arrival, the prehospital responders found Paula comatose. Her vital signs are heart rate of 60 beats/min, respiratory rate of 18 breaths/min, and a blood pressure of 90/60 mm Hg.

   1. What is the most likely problem?

   2. What should the prehospital responder do next?

▼ case progression

The astute prehospital responder performs a quick dextrose test and it shows a reading of 20. He inserts an IV and administers D_{25}. As he is infusing the dextrose, the girl gradually wakes up and declares that she is hungry. The prehospital responders prepare the girl for transport to her home hospital.

▪▪ Diabetes

Diabetes, a common chronic disease, was the sixth leading cause of death in the United States in 1999.[1] Other common endocrine diseases include antidiuretic hormone disorder and thyroid disorders.

Diabetes can result from two different disease processes. Either the body fails to produce insulin or cells resist insulin and therefore cannot metabolize glucose. Insulin is a hormone that "unlocks" the cells of the body, and is needed to convert sugar, starches, and other foods into fuel or energy for the functioning of the body. Without insulin, glucose cannot pass into the body's cells to be burned. If the body can't recog-

nize that glucose is available, it sends out signals to produce and consume more sources of energy. This causes the blood glucose level to rise higher with glucose, eventually overflowing through the kidneys into the urine. When glucose enters the urine, excess water follows and is excreted along with the it. The resulting symptoms are frequent urination, increased thirst, frequent eating, and weight loss. There are two major types of diabetes: type 1 and type 2.

Type 1 Diabetes

Type 1 diabetes, formerly called insulin dependent diabetes mellitus (IDDM) or "juvenile diabetes," affects nearly one in every 400 to 500 children and adolescents under the 20 years of age.[2] In this disease the body does not produce enough insulin and hence the patient is dependent on insulin. Type 1 diabetes represent nearly 5% to 10% of diabetics and tends to run in families.[3] Symptoms of type 1 diabetes typically present in children or young adults, with a peak incidence during puberty, from 10 to 14 years of age. Symptoms are more commonly seen in non-Hispanic whites than in any other race.[3] Depending on the cause, there are two forms of type 1 diabetes.

Immune-mediated diabetes results when the body destroys the cells in the pancreas that produce insulin. Idiopathic type 1 diabetes is the rarer form, and the cause is unknown. However, the management of idiopathic type 1 is the same as immune-mediated diabetes.

Diabetes type 1 can be inherited, can be the result of a self-allergy (or auto-immunity) against cells in the pancreas that make the insulin, or can be caused by a virus or chemical in the food that we eat, which causes damage to the islet cells resulting in an allergic reaction that further damages the islet cells.[1]

Children with type 1 diabetes can lead long and healthy lives if they follow their diabetes treatment plan. This usually includes daily insulin injections (which allow glucose to enter the cells), a specific meal plan (low in carbohydrates), exercise, and regular monitoring of their blood glucose level and urine.

Signs and Symptoms

Hyperglycemia
- Increased thirst
- Increased hunger
- Vomiting
- Abdominal pain
- Dehydration
- Excess urination

Hypoglycemia
- Lightheadedness
- Dizziness
- Vomiting
- Fatigue
- Altered mental status

Type 2 Diabetes

Type 2 diabetes, formerly called adult onset diabetes, accounts for 90% to 95% percent of diabetes.[3] This condition is associated with risk factors such as obesity and lack of physical activity. As the number of overweight and obese children increases, this type of

diabetes is now being diagnosed more frequently, with a predominance found among American Indian, African American, and Hispanic/Latino children and adolescents.[1,2]

Treatment

Children with type 1 diabetes mellitus are on daily doses of insulin to manage their condition. Most children are on a set of doses that are administered in the morning prior to breakfast and in the evening prior to dinner. Their blood glucose is monitored during the day with fingersticks and a glucometer. Although not common, some children may be on a sliding scale. Children with diabetes are on special diets to limit sugars that can cause their blood glucose to fluctuate out of control. They are followed closely by endocrinologists.

Home/Medical Management

- Syringes to administer insulin
- Urine dipsticks to measure glucose and ketones in the urine
- Hemodialysis or peritoneal dialysis if the child is in kidney failure
- Glucometer
- Insulin pump (possibly in adolescents)

Potential medical complications for children with diabetes include ketoacidosis (glucose > 300 combined with ketones in the urine), hyperglycemia (glucose > 300 without ketones in the urine), and hypoglycemia (glucose < 70 and an altered level of consciousness). All of these conditions are life-threatening, but can be prevented or treated at home if caught early enough. When a child is not getting enough insulin or is sick, his or her glucose may get uncontrollably high, and if not treated the child will then produce ketones. The child "spills" glucose in her urine when the blood level gets above 200, and water follows such that the child will have excess urination. This leads to dehydration and ketoacidosis. This can be fatal if left untreated. A diabetic child with hyperglycemic ketoacidosis should be transported to the hospital on IV normal saline and at the hospital should be put on an insulin infusion.

Children with diabetes may become hypoglycemic if they are not eating enough or are ill. Symptoms of hypoglycemia include sweating, tremulousness, feeling of hunger, and altered level of consciousness. These children need sugar right away. If the child is conscious, then giving the child orange juice or candy is helpful. If the child is unconscious, then IV dextrose or glucagon is indicated.

Prehospital Management

BLS Interventions

- Assessment and management of airway, breathing, and circulation
- Provision of oxygen if needed
- Monitor vital signs
- For altered mental status:
  - For diabetic ketoacidosis or hyperglycemia: give oral fluids without sugar if the child is awake and alert and able to tolerate oral fluids
  - For hypoglycemia: give food containing sugar (fruit juice, sugar, candy, honey) if child is conscious or give oral glucose per local protocols

ALS Interventions

- Check glucose level
- Start an IV infusion of 20 cc/kg normal saline

For diabetic ketoacidosis or hyperglycemia:

- Monitor and observe for arrhythmias
- Give only one 20 cc/kg bolus unless cardiovascularly unstable or as instructed by medical control

For hypoglycemia: If serum glucose < 60:

- Give IV dextrose 2–4 cc/kg (0.5 to 1 g/kg) D_{25}
- If less than 30 days old: give 2–4 cc/kg (0.2–0.4 g/kg) D_{10}
- If unable to establish IV access and child is unconscious, give glucagon
  - (< 10 kg) 0.1 mg/kg IM
  - (> 10 kg) 1.0 mg IM

Follow local protocols for drug dosages and administration guideline

---

EMS Tips

Caring for Children With . . .

Diabetes

1. If a child with a history of insulin dependent diabetes (type 1 diabetes) has an altered mental status and blood glucose level cannot be determined, it is not wrong to give IV dextrose or oral glucose.
2. Giving more than one 20-cc/kg fluid bolus to a child in DKA may increase the risk of cerebral edema.
3. Determine when the last insulin injection was given. The onset of regular insulin is about 30 minutes after the injection. The child may begin to experience signs and symptoms of hypoglycemia if he or she does not eat within that 30-minute time frame. However, long-acting insulin (such as Humulin insulin) has an onset of action of 4 to 6 hours.

References

1. Center for Disease Control. Chronic Disease Prevention. The Burden of Chronic Diseases and Their Risk Factors, National and State Perspectives, Diabetes, 2002. Available at: http://www.cdc.gov/nccdphp/burdenbook2002/02_diabetes.htm. Accessed June 2005.
2. Center for Disease Control. Diabetes Public Health Resource, Publications and Products, National Diabetes Fact Sheet. Available at: http://www.cdc.gov/diabetes/pubs/factsheet.htm. Accessed June 2004.
3. American Diabetes Association. Diabetes Facts and Figures. <Online> Available at: http://www.diabetes.org/diabetes-statistics/national-diabetes-fact-sheet.jsp. Accessed June 2005.

Resources

American Diabetes Association. Home Page. Available at: http://www.diabetes.org. Accessed June 2004.
National Institute of Diabetes and Digestive and Kidney Diseases of the National Institutes of Health. Available at: http://www.niddk.nih.gov. Accessed June 2004.

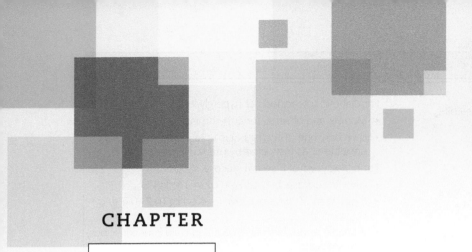

CHAPTER

9 Musculoskeletal Disorders in Children

▶▶▶ case presentation

Emergency medical services responds to a call where an 11-year-old child has fallen out of bed and is now complaining of neck and back pain. The prehospital responders enter the home and immediately attend to the child. As one of the responders reaches for the child's head to take c-spine control, the child's mother yells, "stop!" The mother then reveals that her child has osteogensis imperfecta, also known as brittle bone disease. Further, she states that her son has had over 300 fractures since birth. The child has a condition where C1 and C2 intrude into his brain, and the mother's concern is that a spinal fracture could be lethal.

1. What should be the primary concerns?
2. What should be major considerations with regard to transport of this child?
3. What routine procedures might EMS providers avoid?

▼ case progression

Because this child's bones are very fragile, the EMS providers are extra careful with the child when handling him. As per the mother's request, the crew decides to immobilize this child on a backboard with extra padding. They do not use a collar to immobilize the neck in this child because his neck is very short and the crew feared that they might cause further damage attempting to place the collar. Instead, they securely pad around his neck. When securing the straps they pad underneath each strap. When taking vital signs, they do not take a blood pressure reading to avoid an extremity fracture. The child is awake and alert. His heart rate and respiratory rates are normal for age. They carefully assess neurovascular status of the extremities. They decide to transport this child to his home hospital where he is diagnosed with a thoracic spine fracture.

Osteogenesis Imperfecta

Osteogenesis imperfecta (OI or brittle bone disease) is a genetic disorder characterized by bones that break easily, often due to little or no apparent reason (Figure 9-1). OI is caused by a genetic defect that affects the production of collagen, the major protein of the body's connective tissue. Approximately 20,000 to 50,000 people in the United States are known to have OI.[1]

There are four types of OI. Type I is the most common and mildest form of OI. This is the only type of OI where the collagen structure is normal, but the

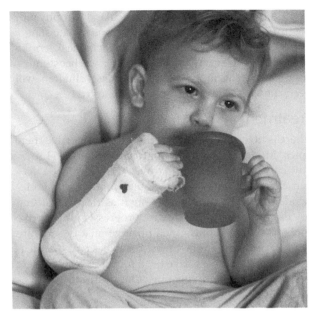

Figure 9-1 Osteogenesis imperfecta.

Home/Medical Management

- Wheelchairs
- Orthopedic devices

Prehospital Management

- Assessment and management of airway, breathing, and circulation
- Place patient on monitor as necessary, but avoid procedures that could cause fractures such as taking a blood pressure
- Insert IVs only if absolutely necessary; avoid intraosseous infusions
- Take extra precautions to avoid further injury, such as securing patient to spine boards securely and with extra padding

amount of collagen in bone is less than normal. All other types of OI have improperly formed collagen. Type II is the most severe form that frequently leads to death at birth or shortly after birth, usually as a result of respiratory problems. Type III OI babies are often born with new and healed fractures. Life expectancy is decreased and few reach adulthood. Their bones continue to easily fracture throughout life. Type IV's severity is between type I and type III.

Signs and Symptoms

- Small stature
- Bones fracture easily
- Possible hearing loss
- Poor muscle development in extremities
- Barrel shaped rib cage
- Spinal curvatures
- Dental problems
- Triangular face

Treatment

There is no cure for OI; however, supportive therapies can prolong and enhance the lives of these children. Treatment is directed toward preventing or controlling the symptoms, maximizing independent mobility, and developing optimal bone mass and strength. This is accomplished through orthopedic devices and surgeries, medications such as steroids, good nutrition, and physical therapy. Most children and adults with OI lead productive and successful lives. There is a variable spectrum of characteristics in children with OI even among children with the same type of OI.

Muscular Dystrophy

Muscular dystrophy is a group of genetic muscle-wasting diseases caused by a flaw in muscle protein genes (Figure 9-2). Muscular dystrophy (MD) is generally inherited, but in some cases no family history of the disease may exist. Progressive weakness and degeneration of the skeletal or voluntary muscles, which control movement, are the main characteristics of MD. The muscles of the heart, involuntary muscles, and other organs are also affected in some forms of MD. Some forms of MD first become apparent in

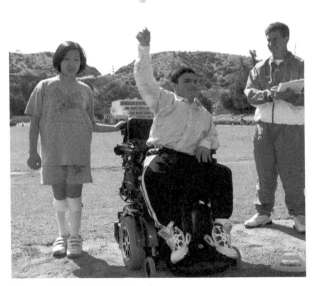

Figure 9-2 Muscular dystrophy.

infancy or childhood while other forms have an onset at older ages.

Duchenne muscular dystrophy is the most common form of muscular dystrophy, occurring in childhood in approximately 1 in 5,000 people.[2] Early signs of DMD usually occur in males between 2 and 6 years of age. Females with the affected gene do not have the actual disease but are carriers of the condition. Initially muscle wasting is limited to the shoulder or pelvic area. Within several years, DMD affects muscles of the upper trunk and arms. Eventually all the major muscle groups are affected. In the late stages of DMD, there is noticeable shortening of muscles and the loss of muscle tissue. There may also be a notable increase in the curvature of the spine.

Some of the late complications of the condition include respiratory infections, <u>cardiomyopathy</u>, deformities, progressive permanent disabilities, and mental impairment in some.

Children with Duchenne's muscular dystrophy may begin to suffer respiratory complications by late school age. These children eventually need mechanical ventilation in order to survive. They will have tracheostomies. As their cardiac muscle weakens, these children will need cardiac medications in order to survive.

Treatment

There is no cure for MD, but there are supportive therapies. Moderate exercise programs and physical therapy can minimize contractures. Orthopedic devices can help maintain and prolong mobility and independence. Respiratory care—such as deep breathing or coughing and as the disease progresses, supportive therapy such as continuous positive airway pressure (CPAP) or ventilators—may be necessary. Medications such as steroids have been found to slow muscle destruction in Duchenne muscular dystrophy.

Home/Medical Management

- Orthopedic devices
- Wheelchairs
- Tracheostomy tubes
- Ventilator
- Feeding tubes
- Cardiac medications if heart failure (Lasix, digoxin)

Potential Medical Problems

Potential medical problems for children with osteogenesis imperfecta include:
- spinal fracture injuring spinal cord
- respiratory distress
- fracture of any extremity, ribs, etc.

Potential medical problems for children with muscular dystrophy include:
- respiratory compromise secondary to weakened respiratory muscles
- cardiomyopathy due to an enlarged, weakened heart muscle

Prehospital Management

BLS Interventions
- Assessment and management of airway, breathing, and circulation
- Provision of oxygen and manual ventilations when needed
- Suction the oral airway or tracheostomy tube as necessary
- Gently stabilize fractured extremities (for a child who has OI, do not use a Hare traction splint to stabilize femur fractures)
- For DNR orders, follow local protocol and contact medical control for guidance

ALS Interventions
- Establish IV access or access central line if indicated
- Infuse a 20 cc/kg normal saline fluid bolus for signs and symptoms of hypoperfusion
- Monitor cardiac status

Signs and Symptoms

- Depends on the type and stage of musculodystrophy
- In early childhood, hypertrophy of calves
- Gower's sign (using hands to get up from sitting position on floor)
- Progressive weakness
- Muscle atrophy
- Progressive paralysis
- Progressive difficulty breathing
- Anorexia

Caring for Children With . . .

Musculoskeletal Diseases

Osteogenesis imperfecta

1. Use extreme caution when moving children with OI. Ask the caregiver for suggestions or assistance.
2. Use extreme caution when taking blood pressure. Compression of the cuff could cause a fracture.
3. Never pick up or pull the child under his or her arms.
4. Never use a Hare traction splint for femur stabilization.
5. Place extra padding between the securing straps and child.
6. Drive cautiously, avoiding sudden jolts that could cause a fracture.

Muscular dystrophy

1. Be careful to support the airway of a child who is in the final stages of MD.
2. The patient may not be able to handle oral secretions due to extreme facial muscle weakness.
3. Use caution when transferring child: he or she may be too weak to provide own support.
4. In the end stages of MD, the child may be very frightened and afraid of dying.
5. During necessary stabilization interventions, provide as much verbal support and comfort as possible.

References

1. Osteogenesis Imperfecta Foundation. About OI, Fast Facts on Osteogenesis Imperfecta. Available at: http://www.oif.org/site/PageServer. Accessed June 2004.
2. Medlineplus. Medline Encyclopedia: Duchenne muscular dystrophy. Available at: http://www.nlm.nih.gov/medlineplus/ency/article/000705.htm. Accessed June 2004.

Resources

National Institute of Arthritis and Musculoskeletal and Skin Diseases (NIAMS), Osteogenesis Imperfecta. Available at: http://www.niams.nih.gov/. Accessed June 2004.

Medline Plus. Health Information, Osteogenesis Imperfecta. Available at: http://www.nlm.nih.gov/medlineplus/osteogenesisimperfecta.html. Accessed June 2004.

Muscular Dystrophy Association. Muscular Dystrophy Association Publications, Facts about Muscular Dystrophy. Available at: http://www.mdausa.org/publications/fa-md-qa.html. Accessed June 2004.

10 General EMS Considerations

1. Treat children with special health care needs as you would any other child. Always assess the ABCs: airway, breathing, and circulation.

2. Use your most valuable resources: the parents or caregivers and the child's home health care provider. The child's caregivers likely know the child better than medical caregivers. Ask for their assistance with specialized equipment. Ask the caregivers or home health care attendant how the child normally acts and feels. This line of questioning will instill confidence in the child's caregivers.

3. Some children with special health care needs have baseline vital signs outside the normal average range for the child's age because of their chronic illness. Also, a medical device (such as a pacemaker or home ventilator) may control vital signs for technology-assisted children. It is important to ask the parents or home health care attendant what the child's "normal" vital signs are. Base your interventions on the child's normal baseline vital signs, not the vital signs that are expected for the child's particular age.

4. Children with special health care needs may have greater difficulty in tolerating respiratory distress or shock than healthy children. Therefore, any medical or traumatic event the child experiences should be considered urgent. Careful and frequent assessments are necessary in order to monitor for subtle changes in the child's condition.

5. Any stressor or illness in a child with special needs experiences can easily increase his or her oxygen consumption, requiring an increase in the child's need for oxygen. Children who are already on home oxygen therapy may need to have their oxygen concentration increased. Those not on home oxygen therapy may need to receive oxygen supplementation.

6. Technology-assisted children may also experience medical emergencies when medical devices on which they depend fail to function. In this situation, prehospital providers must be prepared to use their own equipment in order to support the child's needs.

7. Many children with special health care needs, especially those with spina bifida, have a sensitivity or allergy to latex. Always use latex precautions with these patients. Reactions to latex can range from a localized skin reaction to anaphylaxis.

8. Ask the parents or home health care provider if any special medications or breathing treatments have been given prior to EMS arrival in an effort to correct the child's medical emergency. Monitor for therapeutic and adverse effects from these medications. Base further management and interventions upon treatments previously given at home.

9. Speak quietly and calmly to the child and explain what he or she can expect by using words appropriate for that child's particular developmental

level. This approach will both decrease the child's anxiety and increase cooperation.

10. Recognize that most special needs children respond best with slower movements and firm, secure contact.

11. When leaving the home of a special needs child:
    - Ask the parents for the child's "go bag." This bag contains all of the supplies necessary (and which aren't routinely stocked on a typical BLS or ALS unit) to manage the child's tracheostomy tube and/or feeding tube.

- Ask the parents for the child's daily medical record notebook or medical information form that contains pertinent medical information regarding the child's medical condition, allergies, doctor's names and numbers, medications, therapies, and necessary home support equipment.
- Ensure that any compressed air or oxygen tank in the home is turned off prior to departure.
- Request that the child's direct caregiver accompany the child to the hospital to continue assisting you with the child's care.

EMS Tips

Caring for Children With . . .

Special Health Care Needs

Questions to Ask the Child's Caregiver During an Emergency *

1. Does your child have any including allergies, including allergies to latex?
2. How does your child normally act or respond to you and his or her surroundings?
3. What is your child's normal appearance and color?
4. What is your child's developmental level?
5. Does your child have any vision or hearing problems?
6. Does your child require assistance while walking?
7. How much does your child weigh?
8. What is your child's normal heart rate and respiratory rate?
9. What is your child's normal pulse oximeter reading? Is this on room air or with oxygen?
10. What is your child's baseline heart rhythm?
11. Did today's illness occur gradually or suddenly?
12. What treatments have you administered in order to improve the condition of your child? (i.e., "as needed" medications, oxygen, suction, etc.)
13. Do you have a medical summary card for your child, and if so, may we see it?
14. What hospital do you consider to be your child's home hospital?

*You may not need to ask all of these questions. Ask questions appropriate of the clinical situation.

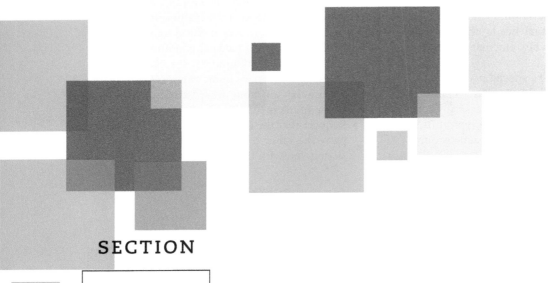

SECTION

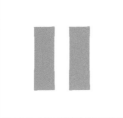

Special Technology

Tracheostomies and Home Ventilation

▶▶▶ case presentation

Mark is a 17-month-old boy born at 27 weeks gestational age. His postnatal course is significant for mechanical ventilation until he was 6 months of age. He was born with respiratory distress syndrome and now has bronchopulmonary dysplasia. Currently, Mark is mechanically ventilated only while asleep. He has a tracheostomy tube. He has a home health care nurse for 8 hours per day while his parents are at work, and his parents manage his equipment for 16 hours per day. He has recently been weaned off of diuretics and for the last two days his family has noted that he is producing more secretions through his tracheostomy tube than usual. Today he has a fever, and the home health care nurse has called 9-1-1 because of a sudden onset of respiratory distress that she is unable to relieve. When paramedics arrive at Mark's home, the home health care nurse meets them at the door. She directs them to the living room where Mark sleeps. Next to his bed are the ventilator and an oxygen tank. The nurse tells the paramedics that she has suctioned Mark's tracheostomy tube several times and he is still in distress. The paramedics note that Mark is breathing quickly and has marked retractions. The pulse oximeter is reading 85%.

1. What are the primary concerns in this child?
2. What should the EMS providers do first?
3. What are the possible problems with this child?

▼ case progression

The primary concern is the adequacy of the airway and breathing in this child. The paramedics attach their manual bag-ventilator to the boy's tracheostomy tube and note that bagging is difficult. The nurse and the paramedics decide that the tube may be obstructed, so the nurse prepares for a tracheostomy tube change. She opens a size 4.5 tracheostomy tube. She places ties through the holes in the wings of the tracheostomy tube. She then quickly places a towel roll under the child's shoulders. She asks one of the paramedics to cut the tracheostomy ties and pull out the tube while she inserts the new tube. The paramedic then attaches the manual bag ventilator to the newly inserted tracheostomy tube and administers several breaths. The pulse oximeter rises and is now 95%. The nurse and the paramedics conclude that Mark did have a mucous plug in his tube, and they begin to prepare Mark for transport. Other concerns in this child include a respiratory infection or an exacerbation of his bronchopulmonary dysplasia. This child has a low respiratory reserve, so seemingly minor infections or asthma-like attacks can be life-threatening. The parents are notified and will meet the crew at the child's home hospital.

Tracheostomy

A tracheostomy is a surgical opening that creates a stoma between the trachea and anterior surface of the neck in order to bypass the upper airway. In most cases an artificial airway, called a tracheostomy tube, is placed through the stoma into the trachea in order to maintain patency of the airway. The indications for a tracheostomy include: to bypass an acute or chronic upper airway obstruction (i.e., tumor or epiglottitis); to provide prolonged assisted breathing support using a ventilator; or to facilitate suctioning by enhancing the ability to remove secretions, such as when the gag or swallow reflexes are ineffective.

Tracheostomy tubes allow long-term medical respiratory support to offset breathing difficulties caused by certain diseases affecting the central nervous system, lungs, or muscles. In many instances, a tracheostomy provides supportive therapy; however, it is not a cure. Examples of medical conditions where a tracheostomy may be necessary include:

- A birth defect (e.g., tracheal atresia, tracheomalacia, cranial-facial anomalies)
- Surgical complications (e.g., accidental damage to the phrenic nerve)
- Trauma (e.g., posttraumatic brain or spinal cord injury)
- A medical condition (e.g., bronchial pulmonary dysplasia, muscular dystrophy)

In most instances, an artificial airway, called a tracheostomy tube, is placed through the stoma to maintain patency of the airway. In some cases, older adolescents and adults may have a well-formed stoma and not require a tracheostomy tube to keep their airway open.

The ability of a child to speak with a tracheostomy tube depends on the type of tube and attachment. In addition, the ability to move air through the upper airway in order to speak may depend on the presence of facial bone abnormalities, or anatomical partial or complete upper airway obstructions due to traumatic injuries or congenital anomalies. A speaker valve can be placed on the tracheostomy tube opening in order to redirect some airflow through the upper airway, thereby allowing the child to speak. A tracheostomy tube, called a fenestrated tracheostomy tube, may have several holes in the curve of the tube below the tube opening that partially redirects airflow through the vocal cords, thus allowing the child to speak.

Tracheostomy tubes come in different sizes and brands. Sizes are marked on the sterile packaging and on the flange, or wings, of each tracheostomy tube. Tube sizes typically range from 00 (for newborns) to 7.0 (for older adolescents). Inner and outer diameters range from 2.5 mm (for infants) to 10.0 mm (for adolescents). Sizing between different brands of tracheostomy tubes can vary greatly. Pay particular attention to the inner and outer diameter sizes of your patient's tracheostomy tube. This information can be found on the box the tube was packaged in or on the flange of the tracheostomy tube. The child's physician, based on physiological and anatomical considerations, determines the brand of tracheostomy tube used. Neonatal tubes are shorter in length than pediatric tubes, even though the inner diameter may be the same. Since neonatal tubes are shorter in length than pediatric tubes, neonatal tubes and pediatric tubes cannot be interchanged. There are various types of tracheostomy tubes. The types used in children depend on the child's size and developmental level. These types include single cannula, the double cannula, fenestrated, and cuffed.

All newborn tracheostomy tubes and most pediatric tubes are single cannula (**Figure 11-1**). A single cannula tube provides a single passage for airflow and suctioning of secretions. There is nothing to keep the stoma open when this tube is removed for changing, so a new tube should be inserted as quickly as possible. Single cannula tubes are placed using a solid plastic insert called an obturator, which helps keep the flexible tracheostomy tube from kinking. The obturator is a solid plastic stylet that is inserted into the tracheostomy tube to guide placement into the stoma during tube insertion. The obturator's rounded distal end helps to prevent tissue damage during tracheostomy tube insertion. The obturator must be removed immediately after insertion to avoid obstructing the airway.

Double cannula tubes are seen in older children (**Figure 11-2**). These tubes have a removable inner cannula that fits inside an outer cannula or sheath.

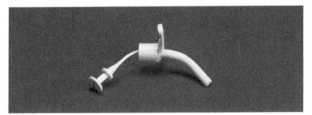

Figure 11-1 Single cannula.

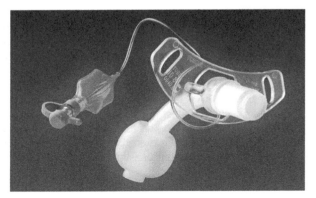

Figure 11-2 Double cannula.

The inner cannula provides a passageway for airflow and removal of secretions, and must be in place for manual or mechanical ventilation. The outer tube remains in the trachea and keeps the stoma open when the inner cannula is removed for cleaning. The double lumen tube also is inserted with the guide of an obturator that, after insertion, is removed and replaced with the inner cannula.

Fenestrated tracheostomy tubes have a hole, or fenestration, in the cephalic portion of the tube that redirects air into the upper airway to allow the child to speak and breathe through the nose and mouth (Figure 11-3). In order to completely redirect the airflow, a decannulation plug is attached to the external opening of the tracheostomy tube. In the event the child is experiencing difficulty breathing through the upper airway, the decannulation plug must be removed to allow airflow through the tracheostomy tube.

Cuffed tracheostomy tubes have a cuff on the end of a tracheostomy tube. This has several purposes. It acts as a seal to eliminate or reduce airflow through the mouth and nose. The inflated cuff also protects the airway from foreign matter. Finally, the cuff gives the tube additional stabilization in the airway.

There are balloon and foam cuffs that can be inflated and deflated. Adult tracheostomy tubes usually have a cuff. Pediatric tracheostomy tubes may have a cuff, depending on the child's airway size and whether or not air leakage has been a problem. Cuffs are not necessary on newborn tracheostomy tubes because the infant's narrow trachea forms a natural cuff or seal around the tube. A cuffed tracheostomy tube has an inner cannula and requires the use of an obturator for insertion.

All tracheostomy tubes, except those made of metal, have a standard external opening so that a manual resuscitator can be attached should the child require assisted ventilation. If the patient has a double cannula tracheostomy tube, the inner cannula must be in place in order for the manual resuscitator to attach onto the tracheostomy opening (Figure 11-4). For metal tracheostomy tubes, if an adapter is not available, the cap of an endotracheal tube can be at-

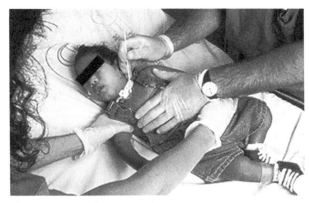
Figure 11-4 Tracheostomy tube.

tached to the resuscitator bag in order to create an appropriate seal.

When transporting a special needs child for an emergency not associated with his or her tracheostomy, the EMS provider should always provide humidified oxygen to prevent secretions from thickening and ultimately plugging the tracheostomy by using one of the following:

- A tracheostomy collar
- A face mask (placed directly over the tracheostomy tube opening)
- A tracheostomy nose over the tracheostomy opening
- Provider-held or in-line nebulized normal saline
- Placement of 1 cc normal saline directly into the tracheostomy tube every 15 minutes in addition to delivering oxygen or using a manual resuscitator when appropriate.

A child with a tracheostomy may have difficulty clearing secretions since the surgical opening in the windpipe bypasses the normal upper airway passages. Other common causes of airway obstruction include improper airway positioning, incorrect insertion of the tracheostomy tube, and mechanical problems with the tracheostomy tube, most commonly a mucous plug (Figure 11-5).

To avoid complications, never force any tube into the stoma. If the stoma or tract site has started to close, possibly from swelling, the child's parents may not have a replacement tracheostomy tube small

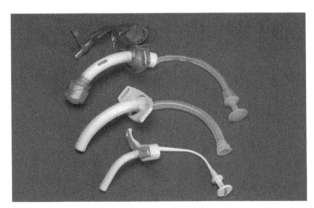
Figure 11-3 Fenestrated tracheostomy tubes.

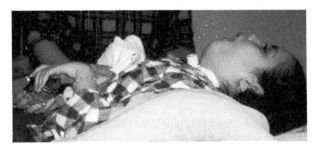
Figure 11-5 Place towel rolls beneath the shoulders to extend the neck in order to assess and manage the tracheostomy tube.

enough to fit through the opening. In this case, use an appropriately sized endotracheal tube to insert into the stoma.

Possible complications from tube reinsertion include:

- Creation of a false lumen or tract
- Subcutaneous air
- Pneumomediastinum
- Pneumothorax
- Bleeding at the insertion site
- Bleeding through the tube
- Right mainstem intubation with endotracheal tube insertion

Signs of Distress

- Nasal flaring, chest wall retractions (with or without abnormal breath sounds)
- Attempts to cough
- Copious secretions noted coming out of the tube
- Faint breath sounds on both sides of the chest despite significant respiratory effort
- Altered mental status
- Lack of chest rise during ventilations
- Cyanosis

EMS Supply Checklist

- Same-size tracheostomy tube "ready to go" with obturator
- One size smaller tracheostomy tube and obturator
- Various sizes of endotracheal tubes (2.5 F–9.0 F)
- Suction catheters (5.0–6.0 F, 8.0 F, 10.0 F, and larger)
- Normal saline bullets for humidification
- Towel to use for shoulder roll
- Sterile gloves, facemask for provider
- Scissors to cut the tracheostomy ties
- Portable oxygen and suctioning
- Monitor
- Manual resuscitator
- Infant, pediatric, and adult face masks
- Water soluble lubrication
- Nebulizer set for delivering humidified oxygen
- Tracheostomy or pediatric facemask
- An oxygen source
- Laryngoscope—blade, handle, bulb, battery
- Parents should have most of these items. Ask the parents if they have a "go bag" or a diaper bag that contains all of the supplies necessary (and which are not routinely stocked in a typical ambulance) to manage their child's tracheostomy tube.

Skill Drill 11-1

Steps for Alleviating Respiratory Distress

1. Place a towel roll under the child's shoulders to hyperextend neck (this will help to open and assess the airway and tracheostomy tube).
2. Make sure the tracheostomy tube is properly in place and the obturator has been removed.
3. If the child has a fenestrated tube, make sure the decannulation plug is removed.
4. If there is no improvement, attempt assisted ventilation through the tracheostomy tube (for ventilator-dependent children, disconnect the tracheostomy tube from the home ventilator and attach a manual resuscitator to the tracheostomy tube).
5. If there is no improvement: after ventilating, if thick secretions are present, inject 1 cc of sterile normal saline into tracheostomy tube and attempt to suction the tube.
6. Use a suction catheter from the patient's supplies, if available. Otherwise, select a suction catheter small enough to pass easily through the child's tracheostomy tube.
7. If using a portable suctioning machine, set it to 100 mm Hg or less.
8. Deliver high-flow oxygen either by placing an oxygen mask directly over the stoma or with manual ventilations. If unable to ventilate, the tracheostomy tube must be changed.
9. Determine proper suction catheter length insertion by measuring the length of the obturator. If the obturator is unavailable, insert the suction catheter approximately 2–3 inches into the tracheostomy tube. Do not use force!
10. Slowly withdraw the catheter, rolling it between the fingers. Apply suction for no more than 10 seconds.
11. If repeated suctioning is needed, oxygenate the child between suction passes.
12. If unable to pass a suction catheter or there is no improvement, an emergency tracheostomy tube change is now necessary!

Skill Drill Tip

Double the inner diameter (ID) size of the tracheostomy tube to determine the most appropriately sized suction catheter to use. For example, a neonatal or pediatric 3.5 tracheostomy tube (3.5 x 2 = 7) would take a size 6 F suction catheter (an 8 F is too large). Formula for determining suction catheter size is:

Tracheostomy tube inner diameter (ID) x 2 = suction catheter size

Skill Drill 11-2

Steps for an Emergency Tracheostomy Tube Change

It is strongly recommended that two people perform this procedure together! BLS providers can assist the caregiver with the following procedure.

1. Ask the parents for a replacement tracheostomy tube.

2. If the child has a cuffed tracheostomy tube, deflate the balloon by connecting a syringe to the valve on the pilot balloon. Draw air out until the pilot balloon collapses. Cutting the pilot balloon will NOT deflate the cuff.

3. If the child has a double cannula tracheostomy tube, remove the inner cannula. If removal of the inner cannula fails to clear the airway, the outer cannula should then be removed.

4. Cut the cloth or Velcro ties that hold the tracheostomy in place.

5. Remove the tracheostomy tube using a slow, outward and downward motion.

6. Gently insert the same size tracheostomy tube, with the obturator in place. Point the curve of the tube downward. Never force the tube!

7. Securely hold the flange (wings) while removing the obturator, ventilate, and assess tube placement to ensure proper placement. Secure tube with tracheostomy ties.

8. If the tube cannot be inserted easily, withdraw it and attempt to pass a smaller-sized tracheostomy tube.

9. If insertion of the smaller tracheostomy tube fails, attempt to insert an endotracheal tube (ETT) no more than 1–2 inches into the opening. Select an endotracheal tube with an inner diameter that is equal to or smaller than the inner diameter of last tracheostomy tube attempted. Be sure to aim the tip of the endotracheal tube downward to prevent tissue damage after passing it through the stoma. If the endotracheal tube has a cuff, inflate it after checking proper placement to help prevent air leakage. Tip: make sure the *outer* diameter of the endotracheal tube is smaller than the outer diameter of the tracheostomy tube most recently attempted.

10. If there is no improvement, or if tracheostomy or endotracheal tube placement is not possible, attempt to ventilate the child by placing a manual resuscitator attached with an infant face mask directly over the stoma (cover the nose and mouth) or over the patient's mouth and nose, using the appropriately sized face mask for the child (cover the stoma to prevent air escape).

11. If ventilation is successful through the nose and mouth, and there is no history of a preexisting upper airway obstruction, the advanced provider can attempt oral endotracheal intubation using an appropriately sized endotracheal tube.

Skill Drill Tip
The tracheostomy tube may be lubricated with water-soluble gel or by dipping it into normal saline.

Skill Drill 11-3
Steps for Using a Suction Catheter as a Guide Wire for Tracheostomy Tube Placement:

1. Thread a small suction catheter that is not connected to suction through the new, lubricated tracheostomy or endotracheal tube until an inch of the catheter has extended past the distal end of the tracheostomy or endotracheal tube.

2. Insert the distal tip of the suction catheter through the stoma and into the trachea, aiming the tip downward.

3. Slide the tracheostomy or endotracheal tube along the suction catheter and through stoma and into the trachea.

4. Withdraw the suction catheter from the tracheostomy or endotracheal tube. Do not let go of the suction catheter at any time before removing it from the tracheostomy or endotracheal tube.

5. Assess for proper placement.

6. Secure airway.

BLS and ALS

EMS Care Tips

Confirm proper placement of the tracheostomy or endotracheal tube by assessing for:
- Equal chest rise and fall
- Equal breath sounds
- Lack of resistance during insertion
- No bleeding at the insertion site
- No bleeding through the tube
- No signs of air in the tissues below the skin (subcutaneous emphysema)
- Improvement in child's color and vital signs

ALS

EMS Care Tips

Resuscitation Drugs Via the Tracheostomy Tube
The following drugs can be given through the tracheostomy tube: Narcan, lidocaine, epinephrine 1:1,000, atropine.
Suggested technique: Dilute drug with 3 to 5 cc of normal saline, instill through a catheter beyond the distal tip of the tracheostomy tube, then ventilate with 100% oxygen and reassess patient.

Medical Devices: Common Problems and Solutions

Device: Tracheostomy
Problem: Obstruction
Action
- Attempt assisted ventilation with high-concentration oxygen
- Attempt to suction
- Change tracheostomy tube
- Ventilate through stoma
- Transport

Device: Tracheostomy
Problem: Dislodged
Action
- Replace tracheostomy
- Provide assisted ventilation with high-concentration oxygen through the stoma
- Transport

Device: Tracheostomy
Problem: Unable to reinsert
Action
- Attempt to place a tracheostomy tube one size smaller
- If attempt fails—attempt to place a similar size endotracheal tube
- If attempt fails—provide assisted ventilation through stoma or through the child's mouth while blocking the stoma

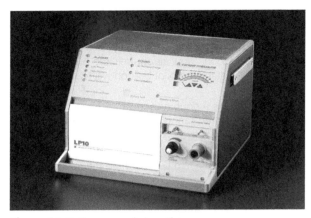

Figure 11-6 Pressure-cycled ventilator.

The common modes of ventilation are synchronized intermittent mechanical ventilation and assist control mode. Synchronized intermittent mechanical ventilation (SIMV) allows the patient to spontaneously breathe—without ventilatory assistance—between the machine delivered breaths. SIMV is designed for patient comfort and will synchronize the ventilator delivered breaths with the patient's breathing effort. SIMV allows the patient to finish expiration before cycling on. Assist control mode allows the patient to initiate spontaneous breaths between the machine-delivered breaths. If the patient's inspiratory effort creates a negative pressure greater than the set level on the breathing effort or sensitivity knob, the ventilator will deliver an extra breath at the set volume on the ventilator.

There are many different models for home ventilators. However, most of them have settings for respiratory rate, tidal volume, FiO_2, peak inspiratory pressure (PIP), and positive end expiratory pressure (PEEP) (see Home Ventilator Settings).

Home Ventilators

Children who depend on home ventilators generally have a problem affecting their respiratory drive or respiratory effort; the ventilator helps these children to breathe. A child with an absent respiratory drive must be supported by a ventilator at all times. In comparison, children who have partial absence of respiratory drive or ineffective respiratory effort may only require occasional support during sleep or times of illness. The ventilator is almost always connected through a tracheostomy tube. Home ventilators are similar to the models used in hospitals. Home ventilator settings can include several different parameters. These are usually determined and set in the hospital and updated as necessary.

There are two types of home ventilators: pressure-cycled ventilators and volume ventilators. Pressure-cycled ventilators are set to deliver a given pressure with each breath (**Figure 11-6**). Volume ventilators are set to deliver a fixed tidal volume with each breath.

Medical Devices

Home Ventilator Settings
- Respiratory Rate—The number of times per minute the ventilator delivers a mechanical breath
- Tidal Volume—The volume of air delivered with each breath
- FiO_2—Percent of oxygen delivered
- Peak Inspiratory Pressure (PIP)—Maximum inspiratory pressure attained during the respiratory cycle
- Positive End Expiratory Pressure (PEEP)—Airway pressure maintained between inspiratory and expiratory phases (prevents alveolar collapse during expiration, decreasing work of reinflation and improving gas exchange)

Home Ventilator Complications

Always ask the parents or home care attendant to help determine the cause of the respiratory problem. They are more familiar with the child's normal appearance and respiratory status and the equipment. Possible causes include: equipment failure involving the ventilator itself, problems with the oxygen supply, obstruction or air leak in the ventilator tubing, obstruction or air leak in the tracheostomy tube, or a medical condition.

There are potential alarms that can alert a care provider about potential problems with a home ventilator. A low pressure/apnea alarm indicates inadequate ventilations or chest rise. Causes include a leak around the tracheostomy or respiratory distress or arrest. Other mechanical causes can include a loose or disconnected circuit, or a leak in the circuit. Interventions include evaluating the patient for signs of respiratory distress (auscultate lung sounds, evaluate color and chest rise and fall), ensuring that all circuit connections are intact and evaluating the tracheostomy tube for leaks, mucous plugs, or dislodgement.

A low pressure alarm indicates a lack of positive pressure required to ventilate. This can occur due to a low battery. Plug the ventilator into an electrical outlet or replace the battery with one that is completely charged.

A high pressure alarm indicates the inability of the ventilator to achieve chest rise and fall due to an obstruction. This can occur because of a plugged or obstructed airway (such as a mucous plug in the tracheostomy tube or bronchospasm) or a blocked circuit (kinks in the ventilator tube). It can also occur when the patient is coughing. Interventions include evaluating the tracheostomy tube and suctioning if needed, treating with bronchodilators if indicated, and checking the circuits.

A power switchover alarm indicates that the unit has switched over from AC power to the internal battery. The "alarm silent" button can be pressed after ensuring that the battery has enough charge to power the ventilator for the time needed. Continue to monitor battery power levels.

A setting error alarm occurs when the ventilator setting is not within equipment capacity (settings have been incorrectly adjusted). In this case, manually ventilate the patient and transport the ventilator and patient to the hospital.

The most common problem results not from the ventilator, but from the equipment necessary to provide a patent airway. Pediatric-size tracheostomy tubes can easily be obstructed with dried secretions that can result in inadequate ventilation. In addition, the ventilator circuitry must be inspected twice daily for moisture and wear, while being changed completely once per week.

Tracheostomy care, such as suctioning, stoma care, and removal of crusty secretions, should be performed by the family or caregiver on a daily basis. Once a week the tracheostomy tube should be removed and replaced with a clean one in order to prevent the skin from adhering to the tube. Good patient hygiene will help reduce the occurrence of tracheitis and pneumonia. If the medical condition continues to deteriorate, observe for progressively worsening signs and symptoms of respiratory distress.

If the child shows signs of respiratory distress or failure and the source of the problem cannot be found and corrected quickly, then the child should be removed from the ventilator and manually ventilated (see **Skill Drill 11-4**).

BLS and ALS

Skill Drill 11-4

Ventilation

Remove the child from the ventilator and provide assisted ventilation using a bag-valve device:

1. Disconnect the ventilator tubing from the tracheostomy.
2. Ask the parents to turn the ventilator off to prevent the alarm from sounding.
3. Attach the bag-valve device to the opening of the tracheostomy tube and begin manual ventilation.
4. Watch and listen for equal chest rise and breath sounds on both sides.
5. If chest rise is shallow, adjust the patient's airway positioning and check to see that the bag-valve device is securely connected to the tracheostomy tube. If chest rise does not improve, assess the tracheostomy tube for obstructions as described earlier here.

Skill Drill Tip
When assessing the airway and breathing of a child with a tracheostomy on a ventilator, always take the child off the ventilator and manually ventilate. This helps the practitioner determine whether the child or the equipment is the cause of the child's respiratory distress.

Signs of Distress

- Decreased chest rise
- Decreased oxygen saturation (a pulse oximeter is required for this measurement)
- Coarse or decreased breath sounds
- Increased respiratory and heart rate
- Intercostal retractions
- Anxiety
- Cyanosis

EMS Supply Checklist

The caregivers should have the necessary supplies to manage the child's tracheostomy tube and ventilator. To manage ventilator emergencies, the prehospital provider will need:

- Monitor
- Sterile gloves and mask
- Portable suction
- 6 F and 8 F suction catheters
- Bag-valve manual ventilator
- Oxygen
- Caregiver supplied tracheostomy tubes
- Endotracheal tubes
- Power source

Special Transport Considerations for the Ventilator-Dependent Child

Whenever possible, the child should be transported on his or her ventilator. This is appropriate as long as the ventilator is functioning properly, the ventilator can be powered, and the child is not experiencing respiratory problems. The parents or home care attendant should be able to provide information on proper transport procedures. If the child requires manual ventilation, it is still important to transport the portable ventilator to the hospital as it may need to be checked for proper functioning.

Proper humidification should be provided during transport to avoid thickening of mucous secretions resulting in tracheal occlusion. If it is not possible to provide humidified oxygen during transport, the child's caregiver or ALS provider can instill 1 cc of normal saline directly into the child's tracheostomy tube prior to transport, then every 15 minutes thereafter. This will keep the airway secretions moist.

The home ventilator can be plugged into a standard 110 VAC wall outlet or into the ambulance inverter. With the unit plugged into a wall outlet, the ventilator can operate indefinitely. The unit is also equipped with an internal battery that is automatically charged when the ventilator is plugged into the 110 VAC power source. The ventilator will automatically switch to internal battery if the unit is disconnected from the wall power source or in the event of an electrical outage. The internal battery can operate the unit for up to one hour, depending on the charge level and ventilator settings. The internal battery should only be used to run the ventilator for short periods of time. In addition, the unit is equipped with a connection port to attach an external 12-volt DC battery (Marine type D cell) or a cable jack connected to the car cigarette lighter. A fully charged 12-volt DC battery will provide an uninterrupted power supply up to an additional 8 hours.

BLS and ALS
EMS Care Tips

- When treating a child with a ventilator, treat the symptoms, not the technology.
- Remember that ventilators are machines and can malfunction.
- In-line nebulizers can be set up using ventilator-assisted respirations.

Medical Devices: Common Problems and Solutions

Device: Home ventilator
Problem: Respiratory distress
Action

- Ask parents to check whether ventilator is functioning properly
- Assist in adjustment of ventilator
- Assess tracheostomy for obstruction
- Remove patient from ventilator and provide assisted ventilation

Bi-level Positive Airway Pressure (BiPAP)

BiPAP may be used on children who have problems with partial airway obstruction or weak respiratory effort. It is intended to augment patient ventilation by supplying pressurized air through a mask (Figure 11-7). It senses the patient's breathing effort by monitoring airflow in the patient circuit and adjusts its output to assist in inhalation or exhalation. This assistance is provided by the administration of two levels of positive pressure. During exhalation, pressure is variably positive or near ambient. The inspiratory level is variably positive and is always higher than the expiratory pressure.

The BiPAP ventilatory support system can operate in the following four modes: spontaneous mode, spontaneous/timed mode, timed mode, and continuous positive airway pressure.

Spontaneous mode occurs when the unit cycles between the inspiratory (IPAP) levels and expiratory (EPAP) levels in response to patient triggering. The patient is in command of the frequency and depth of his breathing. Spontaneous/timed mode occurs when the unit cycles between the IPAP and the EPAP levels in response to patient triggering. If the patient fails to

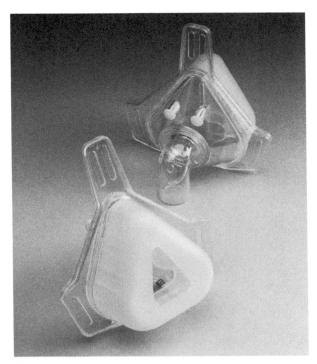

Figure 11-7 BiPAP.

initiate an inspiration, the unit will cycle to IPAP based on a preset interval determined by the synchronized rate (BPM) control. Timed mode occurs when the unit cycles between the IPAP and EPAP levels based solely on the timing intervals as determined by the rate (BPM) and inspiratory time controls. The patient may superimpose spontaneous respirations over the IPAP and EPAP levels. Continuous positive airway pressure (CPAP) occurs with the function selector set either in the IPAP or EPAP position so the pressure will be delivered continuously. The device covers the mouth and nose, or in some cases just the nose, providing constant airway pressure to help maintain adequate respirations and keep the airway from collapsing.

There are special considerations when approaching a child on BiPAP. When a child who requires a BiPAP device experiences a serious illness or trauma, he or she usually has a higher-than-average risk for partial or total airway obstruction. Positive pressure should not exceed 15 cm H_2O, since pressures greater than this may force air into the stomach, increasing the risk for vomiting and aspiration. The BiPAP system is intended to augment patient breathing. It is not intended to provide the total ventilatory requirements of the patient. It must not be used as a life support ventilator.

If the child shows signs of breathing difficulty, ask the care provider whether the child's discomfort is within normal limits for the child or exceeds the child's baseline presentation. If the work of breathing

is abnormal for the child, the prehospital care provider should prepare for transport.

Excessive breathing problems may indicate that the BiPAP device is not working properly. The prehospital care provider should try disconnecting the device to see whether the child's respiratory effort improves. If the child's condition worsens, it may indicate that BiPAP was not the problem, and the device should be reconnected.

The BiPAP device can also be disconnected if it interferes significantly with assessment and interventions. The child will still be able to breathe without BiPAP, but may tire easily. Provide assisted ventilation using manual resuscitation if the child develops breathing problems or becomes obstructed. Consider endotracheal intubation.

Signs of Distress

- Increased breathing rate over baseline
- Nasal flaring
- Subcostal and/or intercostal retractions
- Hypoxia
- Cyanosis

ALS

Skill Drill 11-5
BiPAP Device

1. Remove the child from BiPAP.
2. Provide assisted ventilation using a bag-mask device.
3. Watch and listen for equal chest rise and breath sounds on both sides. If chest rise is shallow, adjust the patient's airway positioning and check to see that the mask is in the appropriate position.
4. If pulse oximetry is available, assess oxygen saturation.
5. If child has persistent respiratory distress, consider intubation of the child's trachea. Transport to the hospital.

Skill Drill Tip
BiPAP is used to relieve obstruction due to sleep apnea or to augment ventilations. It is not to be used for assisted ventilations in children in acute respiratory distress.

EMS Supply Checklist

- Monitor
- Sterile gloves and mask
- Oxygen
- Oxygen masks, nonrebreather masks
- Bag-valve manual ventilator
- Endotracheal tubes

EMS Care Tips

Caring for the Child Requiring Ventilator or CPAP Support

- When in doubt about the function of the ventilator or if the provider is uncomfortable with managing the child on the ventilator, disconnect the ventilator from the child and manually ventilate. The ventilator still needs to accompany the child to the hospital for a respiratory therapist and biomedical engineer to ensure that the machine is functioning properly.

- A child can be transported on CPAP and BiPAP providing his or her respiratory drive is not compromised. CPAP and BiPAP machines are designed to assist or augment patient breathing, NOT to be used as ventilators! If the child has a poor or nonexistent respiratory drive, manual ventilations must be initiated immediately.

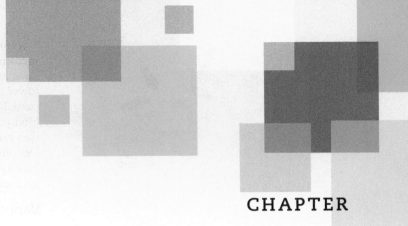

Central Venous Catheters

> ▶▶▶ **case presentation**
>
> Donald is a 7-year-old boy with Hodgkin lymphoma. He receives chemotherapy at home through a central line. Donald was given his chemotherapy treatment this morning at 8:00 AM. Donald's caregiver noticed that Donald had a fever of 101.5°F at 1:00 PM and called 9-1-1. EMS arrives to find that Donald has a pulse of 160 that is weak and thready, a respiratory rate of 30 breaths/min, and capillary refill greater than 3 seconds. He is pale and warm.
>
> 1. What should be done first?
> 2. What is the most likely problem with Donald?

> ▼ case progression
>
> Hodgkin lymphoma is a type of cancer that develops in the lymphatic system, which is part of the body's immune system. Because lymph tissue is located in many parts of the body, Hodgkin lymphoma can start in almost any part of the body. The cancer can spread to almost any organ or tissue, including the liver, bone marrow (the spongy tissue inside the large bones of the body that makes blood cells), and spleen. Children undergoing chemotherapy through a central venous catheter are susceptible to infections. Based on the child's history and the vital signs, Donald has sepsis. Treatment should include assessment of the central line for patency, access of the central line to deliver a fluid bolus at 20 cc/kg, and rapid transport to the nearest appropriate facility.

Central Intravenous Catheters

A <u>central venous catheter (CVC or central line)</u> is a hollow intravenous line that provides access from the outside of the body to a central vein (**Figure 12-1**). The central line can be used to deliver blood products, medications, and nutrition, and is usually placed in children requiring long-term intravenous (IV) access. It also can be used to obtain blood samples. Although it does not eliminate the need for peripheral IV access, it frequently reduces the number of IV sticks required. Placement of a central line is a surgical procedure typically put in by a physician or nurse specialist under local anesthesia. Complications can result from maintenance of the central line as described further in this chapter. In some children central venous lines are for long-term use, such as in children undergoing treatment for leukemia or children with sickle cell disease who need monthly blood transfusions. The types of catheters used include Broviacs and Port-a-Caths®.

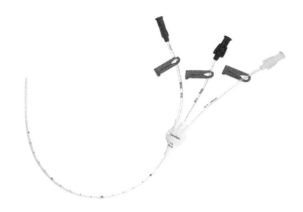

Figure 12-1 Central venous catheters.

Some children need these type of lines for only a few weeks, such as those needing antibiotics for osteomyelitis (bone infection). In these cases, a more temporary type of central line, called a PICC line, is placed (described later in the chapter).

Description of Central Venous Catheters

Types of central venous catheters include nontunneled central venous catheters, tunneled central venous catheters, and implanted vascular access ports. (Table 12-1) Tunneled central venous catheters include Broviac, Hickman, and Groshong catheters. The catheter is inserted through a cut down site into a central vein (usually the external jugular, cephalic, or subclavian) and then advanced to the junction of the superior vena cava and the right atrium. The distal end of the catheter exits from a tunneled subcutaneous space several centimeters from the vein insertion site. Just proximal to the tubing exit is a Dacron cuff that acts as a mechanical barrier to infections and anchors the line in place after a fibrin sheath develops around the cuff 2 weeks after insertion. Exit sites are usually the chest, neck, groin, or arm.

Implanted vascular access port devices include Port-a-Cath®, PAS Port®, and Med-a-Port®. The insertion site and method are the same as for a tunneled central venous catheter. The proximal portion of the catheter consists of a reservoir that is covered with a self-healing rubber septum. This reservoir rests in a subcutaneous pocket in the chest region or between the subcutaneous tissue and muscle fascia, such as in the forearm. The distal tip lies in the superior vena cava. These long-term catheters have no external parts.

Peripherally Inserted Central Venous Catheters (PICC) (Cook and Neo-PICC) are long, flexible silicone catheters usually inserted into the basilic or cephalic vein via the antecubital space. The catheter is advanced into the superior vena cava. Because these catheters are not generally sutured into place, they can be easily dislodged. It is the most common short-term external central venous line (CVL). These catheters are good for patients needing caustic or multiple medications and patients with poor or unreliable venous access. Their use appears to be associated with a lower rate of infection than that associated with other partially implanted external central catheters. Antecubital placement may account, in part, to lower infection rates since the antecubital fossa is less colonized, less oily, and less moist than the neck and groin. A heparinized flush is required once a day in order to maintain patency.

Various Types of Tunneled CVLs

Broviac or Hickman
These are blind-end devices that have a removable cap on the external end of the catheter and a clamp on the tubing distal to the clamp that closes flow to and from the vein. In order to infuse fluids or aspirate blood, the catheter must be unclamped with a syringe or IV tubing secured to the uncapped end. The nature of the external catheter provides an excellent portal of entry directly into the bloodstream for bacteria. Using sterile techniques while working with any central line will help to prevent entry-site or bloodborne infections. These catheters must be flushed with a heparinized solution once per day in order to maintain patency.

Groshong
The Groshong device has a valve near the tip that opens when infusing or drawing back and closes when not in use. This catheter requires flushing only once per week with saline in order to maintain patency.

Implanted Vascular Access Ports

The implanted reservoir port can be seen or felt as a slight bulge in either the upper chest region or forearm. The injection port is self-healing and must be accessed with a noncoring needle that has a solid tip and side hole opening. It is recommended that the injec-

ALS

EMS Care Tips

Peripherally Inserted Central Venous Catheters (PICC)
- Do not place a tourniquet or blood pressure cuff on the same arm as the PICC
- Do not clamp the PICC tubing; clamp the extension tubing
- Do not flush or aspirate from a PICC with less than a 10-cc syringe (smaller size syringes generate too much pressure and can damage the catheter)
- Maximum flow rates are 125 mL/h for 2.0 F catheters and 250 mL/h for catheters > 2.0 F

Table 12-1 CVC Comparisons

	PICC	Tunneled CVC	Implanted Vascular Access Port
Anticoagulant Flush	Daily and after every use	Daily and after each access; Groshong—flushed weekly and after each access with normal saline	Monthly and after each access
Skin Care	As needed	Dressing changes two times a week	None, unless accessed
Infection	Higher—frequent external access	Higher—external access, accessed often	Lower—internally implanted and accessed less often
Body Image	Poorer—easily visible, limited water activities	Poorer—easily visible, limiting with water activities	Better—hidden beneath skin
Accessing Considerations	Standard syringes, IV tubing, no needles, easy external access	Standard syringes and IV tubing, no needles, easy external access	Noncoring needle/connecting tubing, needle insertion through skin

tion needle have a 90° bend; however, there are some noncoring needles that are straight. A standard hypodermic needle will permanently damage the silicone membrane and prevent proper rese aling of the septum when the needle is removed.

General Assessment and Management Considerations

Any child presenting with a central line should be assessed to ensure that the cause of the emergency does not originate from a problem related to the catheter.

This can be accomplished by assessing the child and the central line. Assess the skin at the catheter insertion site for signs of infection. Ensure that the central line is intact. Children who experience problems with central lines should be assessed and treated for respiratory distress and shock. Table 12-2 lists possible causes of central line emergencies along with suggested prehospital management. In all cases, it is highly recommended that local protocols be followed.

If the child depends on the home infusion for the delivery of nutrients, medications, or fluids, the child

Table 12-2 Signs of Distress: Potential Central Line Emergencies and Prehospital Management and Considerations

Type of Emergency	Prehospital Management
External catheter dislodgement	Direct pressure to skin site
Complete catheter dislodgement	Direct pressure to skin site
Damaged catheter	Clamp catheter proximal to the break with a hemostat wrapped in gauze, estimate blood loss
Bleeding at catheter entry site	Direct pressure to entry site, estimate blood loss
Internal bleeding	Direct pressure to site, observe for symptoms of hemopneumothorax
Dislodgement of blood clot	Never force fluids through the catheter! Stop infusion of fluids, clamp catheter
Air embolus	Observe for sudden changes: tachypnea, chest pain, shortness of breath, or loss of consciousness. Clamp system, place child on left side in a head down position, give oxygen.

(continues)

Table 12-2 Signs of Distress: Potential Central Line Emergencies and Prehospital Management and Considerations (continued)	
Type of Emergency	**Prehospital Management**
Fever	Sepsis can quickly develop in immunosuppressed children. Consider fever an emergency. Observe for signs of septic shock.
Reactions from home nutrient or medication infusions	Immediately stop infusion of medications and begin infusion of normal saline. Bring home fluids being infused to the hospital.

should be transported with the fluid infusing through his or her IV pump, if possible. Some children have difficulty tolerating even brief periods of nutrient delivery interruption. The child who depends on hyperalimentation (IV nutrition) whose infusion has been disrupted should be monitored for signs and symptoms of hypoglycemia. Discuss alternative solutions with the child's caregiver and/or medical control if transporting the child while continuing his or her home infusion is a problem. An alternative solution may be to change the IV solution to a solution that is within the ALS provider's protocols. This will give the ALS provider immediate access for medication delivery if needed. In the event the prehospital care provider is BLS, an option would be to request that the child's caregiver monitor the IV medication or fluid infusion en route to the hospital. Again, local protocols must be followed.

ALS providers can access the central line if necessary. However, it is strongly recommended that local protocols are followed and medical control is notified appropriately.

Prehospital use of the implanted venous port is not recommended because the access port is internally implanted and a noncoring needle attached to special connecting tubing is required for proper access.

EMS Supply Checklist

- Syringes (3 cc, 5 cc, 10 cc)
- Normal saline
- Gauze
- Alcohol
- IV tubing
- Catheter clamp

Skill Drill 12-1
Accessing Partially Implanted Central Catheters

1. Do not use the catheter if the child is experiencing any problems with the central line.
2. Prepare equipment (syringes, normal saline, well-primed IV tubing.
3. Wash hands and wear sterile gloves.
4. Scrub the injection cap with alcohol, not povidine iodine.
5. Clamp catheter 3 inches from the cap prior to removing the injection cap.
6. Remove cap and secure a 10-cc or 12-cc syringe filled with 5 cc of normal saline onto the injection port site of the central line.
7. Unclamp catheter and attempt to slowly aspirate 5 cc of blood. (If blood clots are aspirated, immediately clamp catheter. *Do not proceed further.*)
8. Clamp catheter and discard aspirate.
9. Secure a new syringe filled with 10 cc of normal saline, unclamp and slowly infuse 5 to 7 cc into catheter to ensure patency. (If resistance is met, immediately stop procedure and clamp catheter.)
10. Clamp catheters, then remove syringe.
11. Place a well-primed IV line onto injection port, securing with tape.
12. Unclamp the line. Run fluids at a KVO rate, unless the child requires a fluid bolus, and inject medications as necessary.

Skill Drill Tip
Always access central venous catheters under sterile conditions. These lines provide direct access into the central circulation, so it is important to minimize the risk of introduction of bacteria. Many children with central venous catheters (CVCs) are immune suppressed, so infection can be devastating.

EMS Care Tips

Children with Central Lines

- Parents may have appropriate equipment at home, including access needles, to manage central lines.

- If the child is immunosuppressed (ask the parents if the child has a low white blood cell count), providers should wear masks if they have symptoms of a cold or infection. Good handwashing principles must be observed.

- Air embolism can occur unless central line catheters are clamped at all times, except when fluids or medications are being infused or if blood is being aspirated. Air can also enter the catheter if the IV tubing has not been completely purged of "air bubbles."

- A hemopneumothorax can occur as a result of a displaced central venous catheter.

- Insertion of a noncoring needle (a butterfly needle) can result in leakage and loss of the implanted catheter.

Medical Devices: Common Problems and Solutions

Device: Central Intravenous Catheter
Problem: Dislodged or damaged
Action

- Apply direct pressure to stop bleeding
- Clamp or tie exposed catheter to prevent further blood loss
- Assess and treat patient for hemothorax and shock
- Transport

Device: Central Venous Catheter
Problem: Air embolism
Action

- Clamp the line
- Place patient on his or her left side with head down
- Administer high-flow oxygen
- Transport

Device: Central Venous Catheter Site
Problem: Signs of infection at the site
Action

- Treat as a potentially serious infection
- Transport

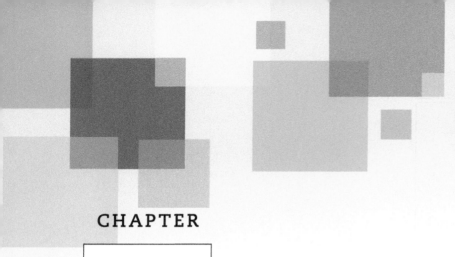

13 Pacemakers

▶▶▶ case presentation

Kadijah is a 13-year-old girl with a congenital heart problem. At the age of 5, she was evaluated for multiple episodes of syncope and was subsequently diagnosed with prolonged QT syndrome. She was noted to have frequent episodes of ventricular tachycardia which led to syncope, and therefore an internal pacemaker with a defibrillator (ICD) was placed. EMS is called to her school by school staff because Kadijah has passed out and they cannot arouse her. Upon arrival, the paramedic notes a pale, listless adolescent with altered mental status. Vital signs are heart rate of 160 beats/min and thready, respiratory rate 20 breaths/min. Blood pressure is not obtainable.

1. What should be the first action?
2. What is the most likely problem with Kadijah?

▼ case progression

Prolonged QT syndrome is a condition where the heart's electrical system does not fire properly, and it can lead to ventricular arrhythmias. Eventually, these episodes can lead to cardiomyopathy and heart failure unless treated. Internal cardiac defibrillators (ICDs) fire when they sense ventricular arrhythmias. ICDs can malfunction, and this should be at the top of your differential diagnosis. The responder's first actions should include assessment of airway, breathing, and circulation. This child should be placed on a monitor to assess her rhythm.

Kadijah is found to be in ventricular tachycardia that is an unstable rhythm. Her ICD has not fired, and therefore she needs to be defibrillated externally. If BLS is there first and the unit has an automatic external defibrillator (AED), this can be applied. Transport to the nearest facility is important. If the responding crew is ALS, then the child should be placed on oxygen, and she should be defibrillated at 2 J/kg or if she is adult size, begin at 200 J. IV access should be obtained, and the child should be transported as soon as possible, preferably to her home hospital if protocol allows.

Internal Pacemakers and Defibrillators

Pacemakers are implanted medical devices that regulate the heart rate. Pacemakers control the heart's pumping activity to keep the heart rate beating at a rate that will adequately maintain perfusion. Some indications for pacemakers include: a heart rate that is so slow that adequate perfusion cannot be maintained, periods when the heart rate is too fast or too slow, a previous cardiac arrest, and heart block especially after open heart surgery.

Pacemakers usually include a generator and leads. The generator contains a battery that supplies the electrical impulse and all the software. Leads are insulated wires that carry the electrical impulse to the heart and carry information about the heart's natural rhythm back to the pulse generator.

There are various types of pacemakers based on how they function. One type senses when a faster heart rate is required and adjusts the rate accordingly. This type usually has a high-end rate limit and a low-end rate limit, allowing the heart rate to increase as needed (with exercise) in order to maintain adequate perfusion. Another type is termed *antiarrhythmia*, which are pacers that sense the heart's natural rhythm and fire when an abnormally fast or slow heart rate is detected.

When treating a child with a pacemaker, the medical provider should ask the following questions:

- What type of heart problem does the child have?
- What rate is the child's underlying rhythm?
- What type of pacemaker does the child have?
- Is the child dependent on the pacemaker?
- If a parent or other care provider is not available, look for a medical alert bracelet or identification tag providing this information.

There are various complications of a pacemaker. One is rapid progression from early shock to late shock. Some pacemakers will not allow the heart rate to increase in response to early shock. If a child with a pacemaker shows signs of shock or has the potential to develop shock, begin treatment for shock and transport immediately. Another complication is pacemaker failure. If the pacemaker fails, the child's heart rate may become too slow to maintain perfusion, which can result in immediate shock and possible arrest. Begin treatment of the ABCs and follow PALS guidelines where appropriate. Transport immediately. A pacemaker can also malfunction. If the child's heart rate is found to be abnormally fast or slow, the pacemaker may be malfunctioning. Begin treatment of the ABCs and follow PALS guidelines where appropriate. Transport immediately. If the pacemaker leads become dislodged, the child's diaphragm may contract, instead of the child's heart muscle, each time the pacemaker fires. Children experiencing this problem usually have periods of fast breathing with no other signs of respiratory distress. The respiratory rate will equal the pacemaker's preset rate. An uncommon problem is that pacemaker leads may break when the child experiences a traumatic injury. Closely monitor a traumatically injured child's heart rate.

Internal Defibrillators

An internal cardiac defibrillator (ICD) or automatic implantable cardiac defibrillator (AICD) is an electronic device implanted under the skin. The purpose of an ICD is to monitor the heart rhythm and slow down or stop excessively fast heart rates that originate in the ventricles. Such rhythms would include ventricular tachycardia and ventricular fibrillation.

The mechanical parts of an AICD include a generator and lead. This generator is a tiny battery-operated electronic device that is located inside a case that monitors and records the heart rhythm, and sends out shocks to convert excessively fast heart rates when needed. The computer also records any shocks that it sends to the heart. A lead (or wire) is attached to the generator and is connected to the heart muscle to monitor the heart rhythm and carry shocks to the heart.

A child who has a history of serious, recurrent arrhythmias with the potential for sudden cardiac arrest would be a candidate for placement of an ICD. The ICD is not a cure for excessively fast life-threatening heart rhythms; however, it can save a life by bringing a rapid heart rate under control.

The medical provider will need to ask the child's caregivers the following questions:

- What is the setting for the child's ICD, or at what heart rate does the ICD fire?
- How many shocks has the child felt?
- Has the child experienced any of the following:
  - Felt more than three shocks in a row?
  - Continuation of unusual symptoms after experiencing a shock?
  - Sensations of dizziness, lightheadedness, palpitations, etc., for a period of time but has felt no shock?

Signs of Distress

- Increased breathing rate over baseline
- Subcostal or intercostal retractions
- Nasal flaring
- Pallor or cyanosis
- Delayed capillary refill/poor perfusion
- Altered mental status

EMS Supply Checklist

- No supplies specific to the pacemakers are needed.
- Resuscitation equipment should be close by in case of impending shock due to pacer failure.
- The child should be placed on a monitor and on oxygen if necessary.

Skill Drill 13-1

1. When there is a condition due to pacemaker failure, treat the underlying condition.
2. If the child is in uncompensated shock due to bradycardia, treat the bradycardia and shock.
3. Manage the child's airway, breathing, and circulation as you would for any other child.
4. Place the child on a monitor and administer oxygen.
5. Obtain IV access. Consider transport to the home hospital. Always follow local EMS protocols.

Skill Drill Tips

Do not become distracted by equipment. The assessment and treatment of children with complex congenital heart disease should progress as with any child. Assessment and management of airway, breathing, and circulation is primary.

BLS and ALS

EMS Care Tips

For Children with Internal Pacemakers and Defibrillators

- The internal pacemaker can easily be felt near the clavicle or in small children in the abdomen.
- Never place defibrillator paddles, "hands off" defibrillating/pacing patches, or AED patches directly over the internal pacemaker or defibrillator generator.
- The battery life for implanted pacemakers and defibrillators is 3 to 5 years.

Medical Devices: Common Problems and Solutions

Device: Pacemaker
Problem: Failure
Action
- Assess heart rate and perfusion
- Treat for shock
- Follow appropriate PALS guidelines
- Transport

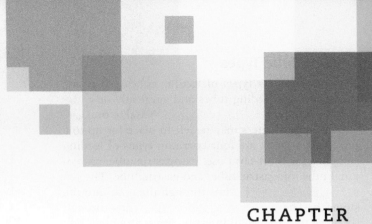

Feeding Catheters

▶▶▶ case presentation

EMS is called to the home of an 11-year-old boy for a complaint of shortness of breath. Jeremy has MRCP (mental retardation/cerebral palsy) and lives at home with his grandmother. He cannot feed himself and therefore has a gastrostomy tube (G-tube) in place for nutrition supplements. His grandmother reports that he has been agitated for the past hour and appears to be having trouble breathing when lying down. EMS assesses Jeremy to find that he has is breathing at 20 breaths/min with some grunting, pulse is 80 beats/min and strong, and capillary refill is 2 seconds. Jeremy is placed on a pulse oximeter and it is found to be 98% in room air.

1. What should be the treatment priorities?

2. What is going on with Jeremy?

▼ case progression

A head-to-toe assessment is performed and the paramedic finds that Jeremy has a distended abdomen. He decompresses the stomach through the patient's G-tube and prepares Jeremy for transport to the hospital. Jeremy's temporary breathing difficulty was due to excess air in his stomach that was pushing on his diaphragm. By decompressing the stomach, the distention was relieved and the pressure on the diaphragm decreased.

Feeding Catheters

A feeding catheter is a tube that is inserted in the nose or through the abdominal wall directly into the stomach. A feeding catheter is designed to manage nutritional needs of children who require supplemental nutrients or who are unable to take food by mouth. In addition, feeding catheters may be used to administer medications. Indications for external tube feedings include:

- Inflammatory bowel disease (Crohn disease, ulcerative colitis)
- Short bowel syndrome
- Coma
- Severe cerebral palsy
- Trauma
- Burns
- Inability to coordinate swallowing
- Failure to thrive
- Diseases interfering with orophayrngeal muscle tone
- Esophageal injuries or anomalies
- The need for a higher calorie intake

Feeding Tube Types

There are various types of feeding tubes. There are nasal and oral feeding tubes and surgically or endoscopically placed feeding catheters. Nasal or oral gastric feeding catheters may be left in place for up to a few weeks. There are four common types of feeding catheters for short-term use: nasogastric tube, nasojejunal tube, orogastric tube, and gastric tube. The nasogastric tube (NGT) runs through the nose into the stomach. The nasojejunal tube (NJT) runs through the nose into the small intestine, presenting less risk of aspiration than a nasogastric tube. The orogastric tube (OGT) runs through the mouth into the stomach; these catheters are used when it is not possible to place a nasal tube.

Gastric feeding catheters are surgically implanted through an external site on the abdomen in children who require catheter feedings for longer periods. Children who have one of these devices have an external button or tube in the abdominal area. A gastrostomy tube (G-tube) is surgically passed through the abdomen wall into the stomach. A Malecot or nonmigrating balloon-tip feeding catheter is placed into the sutured stoma. After the stoma between the gastric and abdominal wall is well formed (at least 3 months) a button device may replace the gastrostomy tube. Percutaneous endoscopic gastrostomy (PEG) is the creation of a percutaneous stoma during an endoscopy.

Gastrostomy Hardware

Gastrostomy tubes may be balloon or mushroom tipped and must have an antimigration device (**Figure 14-1**). The tube's distal end may have a feeding port, medication port, and a balloon inflation port. This tube can be easily vented by unclamping the feeding port. A catheter-tip syringe can be attached to the feeding port to aspirate air from the stomach if necessary. A G-tube button is a skin-level device that has either a balloon or mushroom tip. The button has an antireflux valve. A special adapter is necessary to deliver feedings and to vent or decompress the stomach. Any child experiencing feeding tube difficulties should be transported to the hospital.

Feeding Tube Emergencies and Complications

Potential feeding tube emergencies involving nasogastric or orogastric feeding tubes include: complete catheter dislodgement, partially dislodged catheter, and gastric distention. When one of these complications occurs, assess for aspiration and monitor respiratory status. Assess for dehydration if the child has missed any feedings. Ask the caregiver to check position of the catheter. If position cannot be confirmed, remove the tube (gently pull tube out of the nose/mouth). Connect an appropriately sized syringe to the external

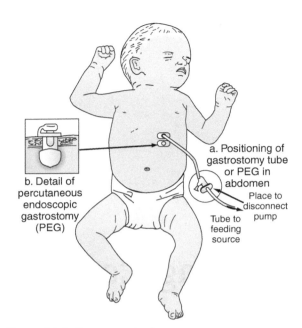

Figure 14-1 Gastrostomy hardware.

a. Positioning of gastrostomy tube or PEG in abdomen

b. Detail of percutaneous endoscopic gastrostomy (PEG)

Place to disconnect pump

Tube to feeding source

opening of the feeding tube, and aspirate until resistance is met. Distention may be a cause of a bowel obstruction or air in the stomach.

Complications involving PEG or gastrostomy tube include: complete catheter dislodgement, irritation or bleeding at the insertion site, gastric contents leaking around catheter, gastric distention, obstructed tube, or broken feeding tube adaptor.

Gastric Distention

The most common cause of gastric distention is air in the stomach. Aggressive manual ventilations can cause gastric distention. In addition, if the child has had a Nissen (a surgical procedure that tightens the cardiac sphincter muscle in order to prevent severe gastric reflux), he or she is unable to burp or vomit. Manually venting (opening) the surgically placed feeding catheter allows air and gastric contents to expel. Gastric contents can be aspirated from both nonsurgically placed and surgically placed gastric tubes by attaching an appropriately sized syringe on the distal tip.

Prehospital Management and Considerations

Assess for dehydration if the child has missed any feeds. Place sterile gauze over the site and apply pressure. The stoma can begin to close in as little as several hours. Emergent reinsertion of the tube in an emergency department is necessary. Cover the site with a sterile dressing and control bleeding. Causes for leakage may include: balloon deflation, coughing, constipation, bowel obstruction, and seizure. After the site is covered with sterile gauze, assess the abdomen. If the tube is still in the stoma, connect the appropriate tubing and syringe to the external opening of feeding tube, and aspirate until resistance is met. Distention may be a cause of bowel obstruction or air in the stomach. Do not force fluids through the tube. The tube needs to be cleared and/or replaced by emergency department personnel. Clamp the tube.

Signs of Distress

- Dry lips and tongue
- Increased heart rate above baseline
- History of no urine output or little urine output in 8 to 12 hours
- Poor perfusion
- Delayed capillary refill
- Cool extremities
- Altered mental status

EMS Supply Checklist

- Monitor
- Sterile gloves and mask
- IVs in pediatric sizes
- IV tubing
- Normal saline
- Gauze
- Syringes: 5 cc, 10 cc, and 20 cc

ALS Skill, but BLS May Assist Caregiver

Skill Drill 14-1
Steps for Decompressing the Stomach

1. Ask parents for appropriate size syringe (or tubing adaptor if the child has a button).
2. Unclamp distal end of tube.
3. Connect syringe, and tubing adaptor if indicated, to the external opening of the tube.
4. Gently and slowly aspirate air and gastric contents until resistance is met.
5. Tube can either then be reclamped or left open. If left open, place the distal end of the tube in a cup below the level of the stomach so contents can drain.

Skill Drill Tip:
Gastric distention is a common problem with feeding tubes. Often leaving the tube unclamped can help, but note that stomach contents can continue to drain.

Tube Dislodgement
Another feeding tube complication is dislodgement of the tube. For G-tube replacement, the medical practi-

tioner should first ask when the tube was first inserted. For tubes that are less than 3 months old, consultation with the physician that performed the procedure is necessary. This is because the track may not be fully formed, and insertion by a practitioner not adept at replacing these tubes may create a false track.

When performing the reinsertion procedure, the practitioner should use a similar size gastrostomy tube. There are different types of tubes including MIC-Key or buttons. Replace with a MIC-Key type of tube. Parents should have an extra tube with them, but if not and your ED does not have G-tubes, then using a Foley catheter to temporarily keep the stoma open is acceptable until definitive placement can occur. Patients should not be discharged home without a definitive G-tube placed. Discussion with the subspecialty service that manages the tube is important for further advice (see Skill Drill 14-2 for gastrostomy tube insertion procedure). If there is a delay in G-tube replacement, then assessment of hydration is important. For the child who cannot take fluids orally, intravenous hydration may need to be considered. Always follow your local protocols before performing any procedure.

ALS, but BLS May Assist Caregiver

Skill Drill 14-2
Steps for Gastrostomy Tube Insertion

1. Obtain same size G-tube and one size smaller available.
2. Check the balloon for leaks by injecting 3 to 5 cc water. Deflate balloon prior to insertion.
3. Lubricate tip with water-soluble gel.
4. Insert gastrostomy tube into stoma.
5. After two to three attempts, if the tube will not pass through the stoma, then attempt procedure with one size smaller tube. Repeat balloon check and lubrication. *Do not force tube.*
6. If the smaller tube will not pass, then attempt to dilate the stoma as follows: Obtain smaller-sized Foley catheters or other catheters available. Insert lubricated smallest size catheter into stoma. Repeat with larger catheters in a stepwise fashion until the appropriate size catheter is able to pass through the stoma. Now pass the appropriately sized gastrostomy tube into stoma.
7. Instruct patient and family to follow up with the practitioner that manages the tube. If insertion of tube is not successful, then the child needs to be transferred for definitive care.

EMS Care Tips

Prehospital Feeding Tube Management

- When preparing for transport, ask the child's caregiver to disconnect the feeding, flush the feeding tube with water, and then clamp the catheter.
- Transport the child sitting up at least 30 degrees to prevent aspiration of gastric contents.
- Always follow your local protocols and seek medical control advice before performing any nonstandard procedures.

Medical Devices: Common Problems and Solutions

Device: Oral or Nasal Feeding Catheter
Problem: Dislodged
Action

- Remove catheter
- Have patient seek medical attention for tube reinsertion

Device: Surgically Placed Feeding Catheter
Problem: Dislodged
Action

- Cover open stoma with gauze
- Transport promptly

Device: Surgically Placed Feeding Catheter
Problem: Abdominal distension or obstruction
Action

- Unclamp tube
- Decompress stomach (aspirate air/fluids)
- Transport

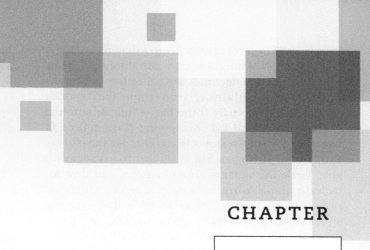

Colostomies

▶▶▶ case presentation

Chaya is a 9-month-old girl who was born with Down syndrome. Soon after birth, Chaya underwent surgery to relieve obstruction of her bowel due to a congenital anomaly associated with her genetic syndrome. She has a colostomy bag in place and is scheduled for reanastomosis of her bowel in the next few months. Chaya's mother called you today because the baby has not been feeding well and has had many full colostomy bags that day.

1. What should be the treatment priorities?
2. What is going on with Chaya?

▼ case progression

Upon arrival a listless and hypotonic child is noted. Chaya has a pulse of 160 beats/min, respiratory rate of 40 breaths/min, and capillary refill time of 3 seconds. The EMS providers conclude that Chaya is dehydrated. With difficulty, IV access is obtained, and she is given a normal saline bolus of 20 cc/kg. Chaya's mother empties the colostomy bag before Chaya is transported to the hospital.

Colostomies

A colostomy is an opening in the abdomen that is formed when the intestine is surgically brought out to the surface and sutured in place, creating a stoma. This procedure allows the digestive system to continue functioning while bypassing any inflamed or damaged bowel. An external bag is placed over the stoma to collect digestive waste matter. The intestines below the colostomy site may not have been removed if there is a possibility of reconnecting the bowel at a later time. Colostomies can be temporary or permanent.

Colostomy Complications

Colostomy complications include dehydration, infection, and bag displacement. Due to an increased risk for dehydration, a child with a colostomy needs to be assessed carefully for clinical signs and symptoms of dehydration and shock, particularly if there is a history of diarrhea or decreased oral intake. Signs of infection at the ostomy site include red, warm, tender skin spreading away from the stoma site. Ask the child or parents if the area is more tender than usual. If the child has signs of infection, transport the child for further evaluation. Sometimes the collection bag breaks or is torn off. Ask the caregiver to empty the bag prior to transport, especially if the bag is full. Be sure the stoma bag is resealed after emptying. If the collection bag that fits over the stoma is missing, ask the parents to apply a replacement bag. If another bag is not available, circle the stoma with moist gauze and then attach any available bag that can serve as a substitute, or place several thicknesses of moist gauze over the stoma until a proper replacement bag is obtained. Another option is to secure a nonrebreather facemask over the stoma. (The nonrebreather bag will collect excreted stool.)

Signs of Distress

Signs of Dehydration
- Increased heart rate above baseline
- Dry lips and tongue
- Poor perfusion
- Delayed capillary refill
- Cool extremities
- Altered mental status

ALS

Skill Drill 15-1

Steps for Addressing Full and Missing Colostomy Bags

1. Ask caregiver to empty and replace bag.
2. Make sure the bag is sealed properly prior to transport.
3. If the colostomy bag breaks, ask caregiver for a replacement. If none is available, encircle the stoma with moist gauze and secure any other type of plastic bag until a definitive bag can be obtained.
4. If no other bag is available, then cover the stoma with a thick stack of moist gauze and replace the bag when child gets to the hospital.

Skill Drill Tip
If a colostomy bag breaks, place a nonrebreather oxygen mask over the site for transport to the hospital.

EMS Supply Checklist

- Caregivers should have the necessary supplies to care for an ostomy.
- If they do not and a replacement bag is needed, apply moist gauze over the stoma for transport or apply a facemask with a nonrebreather over the site as a temporizing measure.
- Always wear gloves when handling a patient's ostomy equipment.

ALS

EMS Care Tips

- Keep the ostomy site moist. Use saline-soaked gauze over the site for transport if ostomy bag is unavailable.
- Be respectful of the child's privacy. Keep the site covered in public.

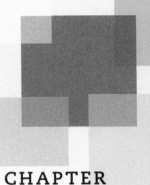

Cerebral Spinal Fluid Shunts

▶▶▶ case presentation

Jordan is a 9-year-old boy with hydrocephalus due to bleeding in the brain during the neonatal period. He has a ventroperitoneal (VP) shunt. Jordan hasn't been feeling like himself over the last few days. He woke up this morning with a headache and has vomited several times. When he became difficult to arouse, his father called 9-1-1. EMS arrives on the scene to find that Jordan has a heart rate of 50 beats/min, respiratory rate of 10 breaths/min, and a blood pressure of 140/90 mm Hg.

1. What are the treatment priorities?
2. What is going on with Jordan?

▼ case progression

Jordan has increased intracranial pressure, which is likely due to a malfunction or obstruction of his VP shunt. The treatment priority is to assess and manage his airway, breathing, and circulation. BLS personnel should strongly consider manual ventilations for the child's hypoventilation, and ALS personnel should consider intubation of the child's trachea. ALS personnel should also consider IV placement without fluid administration. This child should be rapidly transported to the nearest hospital or to his home hospital if EMS protocol allows. The paramedics transport Jordan sitting up, start an IV en route, and call medical control to alert the receiving hospital about Jordan's condition.

Cerebral Spinal Fluid Shunt

A cerebral spinal fluid shunt (CSF shunt) is a catheter that is inserted into the ventricles within the brain, and then threaded under the skin from the skull to the right atrium of the heart or the peritoneum of the abdomen (Figure 16-1). It can be felt as a bump under the skin in the posterior aspect of the head and neck area. It drains excess cerebrospinal fluid that would otherwise build up within the skull.

The purpose of a CSF shunt is to drain excess cerebral spinal fluid from the ventricles in order to maintain normal pressure within the brain. The condition that it treats is hydrocephalus, which is when either too much CSF fluid is produced or there is a blockage to the flow of CSF fluid. This leads to a buildup in the ventricles, creating an increase in intracranial pressure.

A ventriculoperitoneal shunt (VP shunt) originates in the ventricles in the brain and drains into the peritoneal cavity. A ventriculoatrial shunt (VA shunt) originates in the ventricles in the brain and drains into the right atrium.

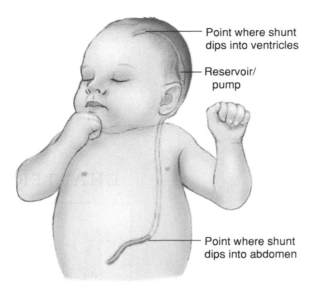

Point where shunt dips into ventricles

Reservoir/ pump

Point where shunt dips into abdomen

Figure 16-1 CSF shunt.

CSF Shunt Complications

CSF shunt complications are always considered an emergency, and the patient should be transported to the emergency department for definitive treatment. Complications include: brain infection; shunt obstruction (resulting in a dangerous buildup of fluid within the skull); shunt malfunction; and peritonitis.

Signs of Distress

- Headache
- Nausea
- Vomiting
- Increased sleep
- Blurred vision
- Irritability
- Loss of coordination
- Alert mental status
- Bradycardia or other arrhythmias
- Fever
- Redness along shunt track
- Apnea
- Seizures
- High-pitched cry
- Full or bulging anterior fontanelle

EMS Supply Checklist

- Monitor
- Oxygen
- Bag-valve manual ventilator
- Endotracheal tubes
- Tape

Prehospital Management

BLS and ALS

Prehospital interventions that may be required include assessment and management of the ABCs, with administration of oxygen and provision of manual ventilations as necessary. For signs of increasing intracranial pressure, ventilate as follows: infants at 35 breaths/min and children at 25 breaths/min. Elevate the head to help decrease intracranial pressure. Consider anticonvulsant medications for seizure activity. Continue to monitor for signs and symptoms of increasing intracranial pressure. Follow PALS guidelines for any arrhythmias.

ALS

EMS Care Tips

For Children with a Cerebral Spinal Fluid Shunt

Ventilating a child with signs and symptoms of increasing intracranial pressure too fast will actually have an adverse effect. Rapidly and dramatically decreasing the CO_2 level causes cerebral vasodilatation and contributes to cerebral edema. It is important that the CO_2 level be slightly lowered to achieve vasoconstriction, thus assisting to potentially decrease cerebral edema. The Pediatric Education for Prehospital Professionals (PEPP) curriculum recommends the following method of ventilation:

- If the patient is exhibiting signs and symptoms of **Cushing's triad** (increasing blood pressure, bradycardia, and irregular/absent respirations):
  - Ventilate the infant at 35 breaths/min.
  - Ventilate the child at 25 breaths/min.
  - Do not manipulate, or "pump," the shunt reservoir, which is usually located at the base of the posterior skull.

Medical Devices: Common Problems and Solutions

Device: CSF Shunt
Problem: Failure or obstruction
Action
- Treat ABCs
- Keep head elevated
- Give anticonvulsants for seizure activity
- Follow appropriate PALS guidelines for arrhythmias

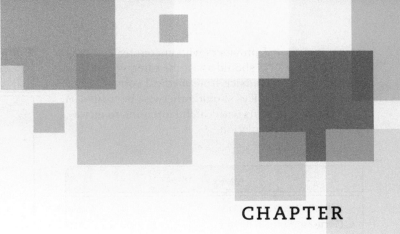

Vagal Nerve Stimulators

▶ ▶ ▶ case presentation

EMS is called to respond for a girl with seizures. Sheila is a 16-year-old girl with epilepsy. She was diagnosed with epilepsy 2 years ago after a serious traumatic brain injury sustained in a motor vehicle crash. She has a new vagal nerve stimulator to control her seizures. She lives with her sister who called 9-1-1 because of repeated seizure activity that did not abate for nearly 10 minutes. EMS arrives to find Sheila on the floor of her bedroom, actively seizing.

1. What are the treatment priorities?
2. Does the presence of a vagal nerve stimulator change your management?

▼ case progression

EMS assesses her airway and breathing. One of the responders places a nonrebreather mask to provide 15 L of oxygen. Her partner starts an IV. Just prior to administering the medication, one of the paramedics asks family members if Sheila has been given any home medications such as rectal Valium. Since she did not get any home medication, one of the responders administers antiseizure medication (such as diazepam, lorazepam, or midazolam) as dictated by local EMS protocols. Sheila needs rapid transport to the nearest emergency department.

◼️◼️ Vagal Nerve Stimulators

The vagal nerve stimulator (VNS) was approved by the Federal Drug Administration (FDA) in 1997 for intractable epilepsy. It is not a commonly encountered device. Intractable epilepsy affects approximately 20% to 30% of patients with seizures. Newer antiepileptic drugs and surgical procedures decrease seizure frequency in a significant number of patients. Even among this group, up to 10% will continue to have disabling seizures. For these patients, VNS provides hope for better seizure control.

The VNS is an implantable device that looks like a pacemaker. It is implanted by a neurosurgeon just under the skin in the chest. In the small number of children who have had VNS placed, most have seen a reduction in seizure frequency of 50%. How the VNS works on the brain is not known. The vagus nerve is a peripheral nerve that leads directly to the brain and it is there that the VNS has an effect.

The VNS is programmed to provide baseline intermittent stimulation of the left vagus nerve. The patient or caretaker activates the device by placing a handheld magnet over the device implanted in the chest. Prehospital providers who encounter a seizing patient with a VNS should assist the caregiver with its activation or seek advice from medical control. Children with VNS devices should otherwise be treated as other seizing patients with careful attention to airway, breathing, and circulation.

Signs of Distress

- Persistent seizure activity
- Decreased breathing rate
- Hypoxia
- Pallor or cyanosis

EMS Supply Checklist

Caregivers should have supplies necessary to manage the vagal nerve stimulator:
- Monitor
- Oxygen
- Bag-valve manual ventilator
- Antiepileptic drugs if allowed by your EMS jurisdiction

ALS
EMS Care Tips

- Treat status epilepticus in a child with VNS as you would any other child with seizures.
- Assist the caregiver with activation of VNS. Assessment and management of the child's airway, breathing, and circulation should be your first priority. Open the child's airway and administer oxygen. Then, if local EMS protocols allow, administer an antiepileptic drug and transport to the hospital.

References

Modified from: Foltin G, Tunik M, Cooper A, et al. *Teaching Resource for Instructors in Prehospital Pediatrics*. The Center for Pediatric Emergency Medicine: New York; 2002.

Resources

Utah Department of Health, Bureau of Emergency Medical Services. *Children with Special Health Care Needs: Technology Assisted Children*. 1998. Book available from EMSC National Clearinghouse, http://www.ems-c.org/products/frameproducts.htm. Accessed February 16, 2004.

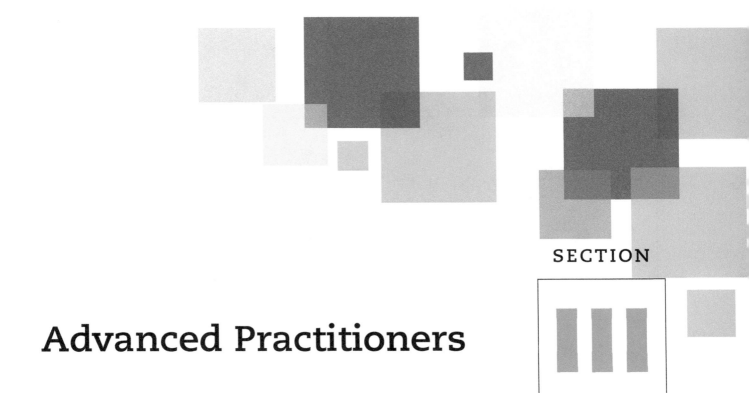

Advanced Practitioners

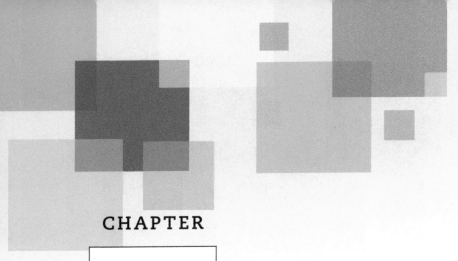

18 Central Venous Catheters and Feeding Catheters

▶▶▶ case presentation

James is a 7-year-old boy with acute lymphocytic leukemia (ALL) who is currently undergoing chemotherapy. His last round of chemotherapy was 4 days prior to his presentation to EMS. The family called 9-1-1 because has a fever and appears ill. He has a Broviac central line through which he gets his chemotherapy.

1. What are the primary concerns?
2. What are the important elements of the history?
3. How should this patient be managed initially?

▼ case progression

The primary concern is that the child could have a serious systemic infection that could lead to shock. It should be assumed that he is immunosuppressed because of his current therapy. Further, he has a foreign body, the Broviac catheter, which can introduce infection directly into his bloodstream. More information can be helpful in his management.

When EMS arrives, they encounter a febrile, pale child. He appears to be breathing fast and his oral temperature is 102°F, his respiratory rate is 40 breaths/min, his heart rate is 160 beats/min, and his blood pressure is 100/60 mm Hg. Equipment that will be needed is prepared (syringes, normal saline, well-primed IV tubing). EMS personnel remember to carefully wash their hands and put on sterile gloves. One of the paramedics scrubs the injection cap with alcohol. He clamps the catheter 3 inches from the cap prior to removing the injection cap. Next, he removes the cap and secures a 10-cc or 12-cc syringe filled with 5 cc of normal saline onto the injection port site of the central line. She then unclamps the catheter and aspirates 5 cc of blood. Next, she reclamps the catheter and discards the aspirate. She secures a new syringe filled with 10 cc of normal saline, unclamps and slowly infuses 5–7 cc of the normal saline into catheter to ensure patency. She clamps the catheter and removes the syringe. She places a well-primed IV line onto injection port, securing with tape and unclamping the line. Her partner gives the child a 20 cc/kg bolus of normal saline through the central line. They prepare the child for transport to his home hospital.

If the child presents directly to the hospital, it is important to recognize that fever in a child with a central line and immune suppression is an emergency. Administering fluids, drawing lab work such as blood counts and cultures, and administering broad-spectrum antibiotics are important initial steps in this child's care. Other important things to consider include the possibility of anemia and thrombocytopenia. This child may also need a blood and/or platelet transfusion as well as antibiotics.

Introduction

Advanced Practitioners

This section is for ALS providers in jurisdictions where these procedures are allowed, nurses, nurse practitioners, and physicians. It comprises a more detailed discussion of central venous lines and feeding tubes with step-by-step procedures on how to manage them. Prehospital emergency responders should only perform procedures allowed by local protocols or with medical control guidance.

Central Intravenous Catheters

Partially Implanted Devices

The external end of a partially implanted catheter may be single, double, or triple lumen, depending on the intended use and the patient's needs. The gauge of the catheter is marked in millimeters on the side of the lumen.

Types of Partially Implanted Devices

Broviac or Hickman

These are blind-end devices that have a removable cap on the external end of the catheter and a clamp on the tubing distal to the clamp that closes flow to and from the vein. In order to infuse fluids or aspirate blood, the catheter must be unclamped with a syringe or IV tubing secured to the uncapped end. The nature of the external catheter provides an excellent portal of entry directly into the bloodstream for bacteria. Using sterile techniques while working with any central line will help to prevent entry site or bloodborne infections. These catheters must be flushed with a heparinized solution once per day in order to maintain patency.

Peripherally Inserted Central Catheters (PICC)

This device is a long, flexible silicone catheter usually inserted into the basilic or cephalic vein via the antecubital space. The catheter is advanced into the superior vena cava. It is the most common short-term external CVL. These catheters are not generally sutured into place. Their use appears to be associated with a lower rate of infection than that associated with other partially implanted external central catheters. Antecubital placement may account, in part, to lower infection rates. The antecubital fossa is less colonized, less oily, and less moist than the neck and groin. A heparinized flush is required once per day in order to maintain patency.

Totally Implanted Devices

The implanted reservoir port can be seen or felt as a slight bulge in either the upper chest region or forearm. The injection port is self-healing and must be accessed with a noncoring needle that has a solid tip and side hole opening. It is recommended that this injection needle has a 90 degree bend; however, there are some noncoring needles that are straight. A standard hypodermic needle will permanently damage the silicone membrane and prevent proper resealing of the septum when the needle is removed. Totally implanted devices may be referred to as a Port-a-Cath®, Mediport®, or PAS Port®.

Central Line Comparisons

PICC lines require anticoagulant flushing daily and with each access. Skin care is as needed. Infection rates tend to be higher than with other catheters because these lines are external and are accessed often. These types are catheters are not good for adolescents who are sensitive to body image. PICC lines are readily visible and swimming is contraindicated. PICC lines are best for short-term needs (weeks). Equipment needs include standard syringes and IV tubing, but needles are not necessary, thus making external access easy.

Partially implanted lines such as the Groshong need normal saline flushing weekly and with each access. Other types of lines need anticoagulant flushes daily and with each access. Skin care includes dressing changes twice per week. Infection rates tend to be higher than with other types of catheters because these are external lines that are accessed often. These lines are not ideal for adolescents who are sensitive to body image. Swimming is contraindicated. These types of lines are best for short-term needs (months). Equipment needed includes standard syringes and IV tubing. No needles are necessary, making access easy.

Completely implanted devices need anticoagulant flushing monthly and with every access. No special skin care is needed. Infection rates tend to be low as these are internal, not exposed to the outside, and are accessed less often. These are best for adolescents who have body image issues because these devices are hidden. These are best for long-term needs (years). Special noncoring needles are needed for access as well as connection tubing. The needle is inserted through the skin, so families often ask for EMLA (eutectic mixture of lidocaine analogs) cream prior to access.

Potential Central Line Emergencies and Physician Management/Considerations

If there is external catheter dislodgement, then the health care practitioner should apply direct pressure to skin site and clamp the line near the exit site. Place a peripheral IV if necessary to continue fluids and medications. Consider a chest x-ray to locate the distal end of catheter. Also consider a dye study to determine location of catheter tip. Obtain a surgical consultation for catheter replacement.

For complete catheter dislodgement, apply direct pressure to skin site. Place a peripheral IV to continue necessary fluids and medications, and obtain a surgical consultation to determine disposition and need for a new central catheter.

For a damaged catheter, clamp catheter proximal to the break with a hemostat wrapped in gauze. Estimate blood loss. Observe for symptoms of air embolus. If PICC line, consider complete removal. For other partially implanted lines, repair catheter if more than 2 inches of the line exit from the skin.

For bleeding at catheter entry site, apply direct pressure to entry site. Estimate blood loss. Place a peripheral IV to continue necessary fluids and medications. Consider a chest x-ray to locate the distal end of catheter. Also consider a dye study to determine location of catheter tip. Obtain surgical consultation.

For internal bleeding, apply direct pressure to site. Observe for symptoms of hemopneumothorax. Place a peripheral IV to continue necessary fluids and medications. Consider a chest x-ray to locate distal end of catheter. Consider a dye study to determine location of catheter tip. Obtain surgical consultation.

For catheter occlusion, with problems withdrawing blood, try placing the child in various positions (arms high, laying supine, etc.). Attempt to gently aspirate the clot using a 10-cc syringe half filled with normal saline placed directly onto the male Leur lock of the catheter. Consider using a fibrinolytic agent.

For dislodgement of blood clot, never force fluids through the catheter because pulmonary embolism may result. Observe for tachycardia, tachypnea, hypoxemia, and chest pain (signs and symptoms of pulmonary embolism). Immediately stop infusion of fluids. Clamp the catheter.

For concern about air embolus, observe for sudden changes: tachypnea, chest pain, shortness of breath, or loss of consciousness. Clamp the system, place child on left side in a head down position, administer oxygen.

For fever and central venous catheter, consider the patient bacteremic or septicemic until proven otherwise. Sepsis can develop quickly in immunosuppressed children. Evaluate for source of infection. Begin broad spectrum antibiotics. Admit the child to the hospital for antibiotic therapy until culture results are known in 48 to 72 hours.

For reactions from home nutrient or medication infusions, immediately stop the infusion of medications and begin infusion of normal saline. Treat signs of allergic reaction with Benadryl, steroids, and subcutaneous injections of 1:1,000 epinephrine if symptoms are severe.

ALS

Skill Drill 18-1

Accessing Partially Implanted Central Catheters

1. Do not use the catheter if the child is experiencing any problems with the central line.

2. Prepare equipment (syringes, normal saline, well-primed IV tubing).
3. Wash hands and wear sterile gloves.
4. Scrub the injection cap with alcohol, not povidine iodine.
5. Clamp catheter 3 inches from the cap prior to removing the injection cap.
6. Remove cap and secure a 10-cc or 12-cc syringe filled with 5 cc of normal saline onto the injection port site of the central line.
7. Unclamp catheter and attempt to slowly aspirate 5 cc of blood. (If blood clots are aspirated, STOP; immediately clamp catheter, do not proceed further.) Clamp catheter and discard aspirate.
8. Secure a new syringe filled with 10 cc of normal saline, unclamp and slowly infuse 5 to 7 cc into catheter to ensure patency. (If resistance is met, immediately stop procedure and clamp catheter.)
9. Clamp catheter and then remove syringe.
10. Place a well-primed IV line onto injection port, securing with tape.
11. Unclamp the line.
12. Run fluids at a KVO rate, unless the child requires a fluid bolus, and inject medications as necessary.
13. If line is used only to draw a blood sample, flush with heparin prior to removing syringe from catheter tip. Clamp catheter after heparinizing line.

ALS

Skill Drill 18-2

Accessing Completely Implanted Catheters

1. Place EMLA cream on skin over injection port for 60 minutes.
2. Wipe away EMLA cream.
3. Prepare equipment (syringes, normal saline, well-primed IV tubing).
4. Wash hands and don sterile gloves and facemask.
5. Palpate reservoir and scrub overlying skin with povidine iodine, washing in a circular motion.
6. Attach a 10-cc syringe filled with saline to a T-connector, and then flush saline through tubing.
7. Attach this extension set to a Huber or other noncoring needle.
8. Flush needle with saline to remove any air.
9. Clamp extension tubing closed.
10. Don a new pair of sterile gloves.
11. Locate center of port, and stabilize with thumb and index finger.
12. Slowly but firmly insert needle through center of port to back of reservoir.
13. Unclamp extension tubing and inject 2 cc of saline into reservoir.
14. If resistance is met, do not force. Gently attempt to aspirate blood. If unable to aspirate blood or flush line, clamp extension set and remove needle from port.

15. If no resistance is met injecting saline, aspirate fluid back into syringe and check for blood return. (If blood clots are aspirated *do not* proceed further.) Clamp catheter and discard aspirate.

16. Secure a new syringe filled with 10 cc of normal saline, unclamp, and slowly infuse 5 to 7 cc into catheter to ensure patency. (If resistance is met, immediately stop procedure and clamp catheter.)

17. Clamp catheter, then remove syringe.

18. Place a well-primed IV line onto extension port, securing with tape.

19. Unclamp the line.

20. Run fluids at a KVO rate, unless the child requires a fluid bolus, and inject medications as necessary.

21. Place dressing over access site.

22. If line is used only to draw a blood sample, flush with heparin prior to removing needle from reservoir.

Alteplase (tPA) for Venous Catheter Occlusion

Alteplase (1 mg/mL) instilled into a central catheter in 1 to 2 doses may be used to restore patency to catheters, which have been occluded by blood or fibrin. Alteplase may be used to restore blood flow through a Broviac, Port-a-Cath, PICC, or temporary central venous catheter. Alteplase is a tissue plasminogen activator (tPA) produced by recombinant DNA. It is a sterile, purified glycoprotein of 527 amino acids. It is synthesized using the complementary DNA for natural human tissue-type plasminogen activator obtained from a human cell culture.

Prior to administration of tPA, the health care practitioner should be cognizant of potential problems with the central catheter, such as difficulty with administration. The catheter tip may be against the vessel wall. A change in position may reverse this. Have patient lie on the left side and take a deep breath or raise both arms over the head. A small thrombus can act as a flap valve across the lumen of the catheter tip. Gently irrigate with normal saline to clear the lumen before attempting aspiration. Never force solution through the catheter when resistance is encountered. The needle of a Port-a-Cath may be dislodged or occluded. Press firmly on the needle to move it to the back wall of the diaphragm. If unsuccessful, remove the needle and flush for patency. Attempt to re-access the patient one time. Determine whether the occlusion is most likely caused by blood, medication precipitate, or lipid sludge. If the most likely cause of the occlusion is a blood or fibrin clot, a physician will order the prescribed dose and volume of alteplase after verification of the occlusion. A trained registered nurse or physician will administer alteplase as outlined in the procedure in Skill Drill 18-3.

Skill Drill 18-3
Clearing Occluded Catheters

1. Wash hands.

2. Explain procedure to child/parents.

3. Thaw 2 mg/2 mL frozen vial of alteplase. Roll vial between your hands to thaw.

4. Withdraw alteplase into syringe.

5. Attach a 10-mL empty syringe to occluded catheter and aspirate air/fluid to create a vacuum; clamp catheter while maintaining a vacuum.

6. Attach alteplase syringe to catheter and unclamp.

7. Slowly instill solution, filling catheter.

8. Clamp the catheter and wait 30 minutes to 1 or 2 hours.

9. Withdraw 1 to 3 mL blood. The volume of blood withdrawn should be a little more than the amount of medication infused. *Discard this blood.*

10. If unsuccessful, wait 30 minutes and administer alteplase one more time using the same procedure.

11. If unsuccessful the second time, evaluate other treatment options. Consult with the attending physician.

12. When patentcy is restored, after aspirating 1 to 3 mL blood, flush the catheter with 2 to 10 mL of normal saline.

13. Heparinize the catheter per protocol or reconnect the IV solution.

14. Document any pertinent observations in the progress notes and each dose on the medical administration record.

Skill Drill Tips

It is best to use alteplase as soon as possible. Use thawed vial within 8 hours of removal from freezer. Do not shake solution. Do not dilute. The volume of alteplase to instill is equal to the internal volume of the catheter. If you do not know the catheter volume, the following may be used as a guide: Broviac: 0.2–0.4 mL in 1-mL syringe, Port-a-Cath: 2 mL in 3-mL syringe, PICC: 0.3–0.5 mL in 1-mL syringe, Neonatal CVL: 0.3 mL in 1-mL syringe, Child CVL: 1 mL in 3-mL syringe, Adult CVL: 1–3 mL in 3-mL syringe.

Do not force medication into the catheter. Administer alteplase into each occluded lumen. Put an altsplase (tPA) label on the tubing so no one will instill the medication by mistake. Observe catheter for breakage/leakage. Avoid administering alteplase systemically. Pull medication from catheter using a turbulant (start/stop) technique to clear catheter completely. If occlusion occurs during medication administration or while receiving total parenteral nutrition, consider precipitation instead of blood and fibrin clot. Always use a positive-pressure flush technique.

Feeding Catheters

External tube feedings involve any form of nutrition delivered to the gastrointestinal tract by artificial means.

Medical Devices: Common Problems and Solutions

Troubleshooting

Potential Problems

Nausea, vomiting, cramping and/or diarrhea

Possible Causation

- Too rapid feeding
- Feeding too cold
- Spoiled formula or a change in formula

Actions

- Increase feeding time
- Insure feeding is at room temperature

Potential Problem

Leakage of stomach contents

Possible Causation

- Mechanical
  - Broken or sticking valve
  - Incorrectly positioned tube wedged into the gastric mucosa
  - Balloon not inflated properly
- Organic
  - Increased volume of feeding (too much gas or formula)
  - Constipation
  - Ileus
  - Pneumonia (from coughing)
  - Seizures

Actions

- Place insertion obturator, decompression tube, or 8–10 F suction catheter into shaft of button so it moves the flex valve. Antireflux valve makes popping sound when it moves back into closed position.
- Ensure balloon is fully inflated
- Check stomach residual, readjust method of feedings as appropriate
- Evaluate for other organic causes and treat accordingly

Potential Problem

Blockage of the button

Possible Causation

- Feeding or medications too thick or remain in shaft too long

Actions

- Flush button with 5–10 cc of tap water after using

- Use thin solutions with well-crushed meds
- Use insertion obturator or 8–10 F suction catheter to gently try to push the plug through

Potential Problem

Accidental removal of button

Possible Causation

- Vigorous pulling on the button
- Spontaneous deflation of the gastrostomy balloon

Actions

- Insert gastrostomy tube to keep stoma open
- As a last resort, a Foley catheter with an antimigration device may be inserted into the stoma. Tube must be securely taped in place. Immediately transport to tertiary hospital for button replacement.
- Button length may be too long

Potential Problem

Stoma site irritation

- Maceration due to moisture
- Gastric acid burn from leakage of gastric contents
- Purulent mucous

Possible Causation

- Regular cleaning not effective
- Incomplete drying
- Feeding spillage with incomplete cleaning
- Leakage of gastric contents from or around tube
- Excessive granulation tissue

Actions

- Button length may be too short
- Do not use occlusive dressing, gauze, tape, or creams
- Rotate button 360° once per day
- Clean site daily with soap and water
- Clean site with 1/3-strength hydrogen peroxide if irritated
- Consider using a skin barrier cream and H2 blocker for gastric burns.

Potential Problem

Balloon leaks or ruptures

Possible Causation

- Silicone balloons generally last about 3 months; however, life of balloon may vary

Actions

Replace gastrostomy button

Tube feedings should be considered when the patient has either impaired or insufficient oral intake, has a functional gut, and a safe method of access. An absolute contraindication for external tube feedings is anatomic obstruction.

Nasogastric Tube Feedings (NG)

NG tube feedings should be considered for short-term use (< 30 days). NG tubes should be placed with ex-treme caution in patients with an altered level of consciousness. All patients should be assessed for proper placement prior to beginning feedings. NG tubes are for short-term use, with the average life of the tube being 10 days. Feedings may be delivered by bolus, gravity, or pump-controlled techniques. The preferred method depends on the patient's needs and tolerance of the method of feeding. Nasogastric feeding catheters should be made out of polyurethane or silicone. If the catheter is made of polyvinyl chloride, it should be changed every 72 hours since these tubes become stiff and may crack and cause perforation.

Gastrostomy, Jejunostomy, or Gastrojejunostomy Tubes (G-tubes, J-tubes, G-J tubes)

G-tubes or J-tubes should be considered when a patient will require prolonged tube feeding (> 30 days). Available techniques for placement of these tubes include: percutaneous gastrostomy (endoscopic [PEG] or radiological); percutaneous jejunostomy (endoscopic [PJG] or radiological); percutaneous gastrojejunostomy ([PEG/J] endoscopic or radiological); surgical gastrostomy; or surgical jejunostomy.

Types of Gastrostomy Devices
Gastrostomy Tubes

There are several types of G-tubes, and they are often called by their manufacturer's names. The Malencot has a feeding port, and the proximal end of tube is mushroom tipped. A balloon-ended type, such as a Foley catheter, has a feeding port and a balloon inflation port. An antimigration device must be on this tube.

It is important to note that these tubes do not have an antireflux valve. They can be easily vented simply by uncapping the feeding port. A common type of G-tube is the MIC-G® tube, which has shaft lengths from 0.8 to 4.5 cm. It has a port that can be closed when not in use. This tube does not have an antireflux valve. Printed marks on the shaft assist in proper tube positioning.

Buttons

A button is another type of G-tube. The proximal end may either be rigid, mushroom tipped, or balloon type. Button tubes have an antireflux valve that requires special adapter tubing to access. It is important to note that gastrostomy buttons should not be inserted until firm adhesions between the gastric and abdominal wall are established in order to prevent gastric separation. The recommended amount of time from surgical placement of gastrostomy tube until placement of G-tube button is at least 3 months, but it may be longer if the patient is malnourished or on steroids. Also, the gastrostomy button must be rotated 360° once a day to prevent entrapment into the gastric mucosa.

Examples of types of gastrostomy buttons include the MIC-Key Low Profile®, which has a safety plug, proximal anti-reflux valve, medication port, and an external extension set that locks, thus preventing accidental disconnection. It sits at 90° to the skin and is manufactured by Medical Innovations Corporation (Ballard). The Ross-Abbott Stomate Low-Profile Gastrostomy has a safety plug, anti-reflux valve, and a Y-port connector with a right angle adapter. The Bard Button has a safety plug, anti-reflux valve, and venting (decompression) via a special additional venting tube. The Corpak Low-Profile Gastrostomy Device has a safety plug, anti-reflux valve, and additional vent tubing.

Complications of Gastrostomy Devices

The most common reasons for ER visits for patients with feeding catheters include: gastrostomy tube or button has come out, tube deterioration, a malfunctioning tube, a blocked tube due to formula or medication, a blocked tube due to mechanical twisting or kinking, the stoma site is has yellowish purulent drainage and gastric mucosa is coming out of the stoma, there is bleeding at the stoma site, there is pain at the stoma site, the PEG cannot be rotated (i.e., the PEG is no longer properly positioned).

Questions to ask parents prior to replacing feeding catheter include: What type of procedure was done in order to place the feeding catheter; if it was surgical placement, was a Nissen done or any other antireflux measure taken? And importantly, when was the surgery done? When and how the surgery was done determines what type of device can be placed into the stoma site. If surgery was > 4 months prior, any knowledgeable physician can attempt to replace the feeding catheter. If surgery was < 30 days, the tube needs to be replaced by a surgeon or gastroenterologist.

Medical Devices: Common Problems and Solutions

Troubleshooting

Measures to take if stoma has begun to close:
- Dilate the stoma site up by using soft catheters such as Robnel or smaller Foley catheters.
- Metal Hegar dilators should only be used by a surgeon or a gastroenterologist while the child is sedated.
- *Never dilate recently placed tracts!*

ALS

Skill Drill 18-4

Steps for Inserting the MIC-Key (Button) Skin-Level Feeding Tube

1. Lubricate the tip of the new MIC-Key with a water-soluble agent.
2. Gently guide the new tube into the stoma. Insert the tube all the way until the MIC-Key is flat against the skin.

3. Hold the tube in place and inflate the balloon with sterile water, distilled water, or normal saline. Do not use air. Never fill the balloon with more than 5 cc of fluid. For infants, instill no more than 2–3 cc.

4. Position the balloon against the stomach wall by pulling the MIC-Key up and away very gently until it stops.

5. Wipe away fluid or lubricant from the tube and stoma.

6. Check the tube for correct placement by inserting an extension set into the feeding port and listening for air sounds when air is injected into the stomach with a syringe. Tube placement should also be confirmed by aspirating stomach contents.

ALS

Skill Drill 18-5

Steps for Inserting a Gastrostomy Feeding Tube

1. Choose the appropriate size replacement tube.

2. It is desirable that the replacement tube be of the same type and size as the original tube.

3. If a balloon-tipped Foley catheter must be used, it should only be substituted as a temporizing measure only. It must have an antimigration device and be securely taped into place.

4. Consider conscious sedation.

5. With balloon-tipped tubes, balloon integrity should be checked. Inject 5 cc of water into the short tube, or balloon injection port, to blow up balloon.

6. Observe for leakage.

7. If balloon remains full for 2 minutes, remove water from balloon and proceed.

8. Collapsible wing or mushroom-tipped catheters should be checked. Ensure that the stylet or obturator properly distends the distal tip so that it is narrowed prior to passing through the stoma.

9. If gastrostomy device must be removed, the following must be considered: Detach any clamps or external sources of stabilization. If device has a balloon tip, aspirate fluid. If device is mushroom tipped, insert stylet or obturator into the tube to extend the distal tip within the stomach wall.

10. Moisten the tip of the tube, coat the stoma site liberally with water-soluble lubricant, and gently insert the G-tube through the stoma into the stomach.

11. Hold new catheter perpendicular to the skin.

12. Gently insert with continuous pressure into the stoma site, and steadily advance for several centimeters until well inside the stomach.

13. Remove the obturator or stylet, if used.

14. Inflate the balloon, if present, with 3–5 cc of water or saline.

15. Observe for gastric leakage around stoma. If the stoma leaks, increase the balloon volume by 2 cc. Repeat this step until the leak stops. Do not exceed 5 cc of fluid volume inside the balloon.

16. Check for correct tube position and patency.

17. Aspirate for gastric contents.

18. Instill 10 to 15 cc of air auscultating for borborygami to confirm placement.

19. If unable to confirm tube placement, radiographic studies are indicated.

20. Secure the tube (use tape or sutures).

21. Clamp or close the distal tube opening.

22. Begin tube feedings only after ensuring proper tube placement.

ALS

Skill Drill 18-6

Jejunostomy Tube Replacement

1. The specialist who originally placed the tube should do the reinsertion.

2. A temporary solution is to have an experienced radiologist replace the tube under fluoroscopy.

3. Blindly passing the weighted nasoduodenal tube should not be attempted.

Medical Devices: Common Problems and Solutions

Troubleshooting

Potential Problems

- Accidental formation of a false track
- Separation of the stomach wall from the peritoneal wall resulting in peritoneal insertion of the tube (installation of fluid there can cause chemical peritonitis)

Causation

- Improper insertion of the gastrostomy tube
- Migration of the tube
- Improperly secured tube

Action

- Do not use the tube for feedings.
- Remove the tube and reinsert.
- Perform radiographic dye study to ensure proper placement of tip in stomach prior to use. (Inject a small amount of radioopaque dye and then take x-ray.)

Potential Problem

- Replacement tube not advanced far enough, leaving the distal tip in the fistula as opposed to the stomach lumen

Causation

- Improper insertion of tube

Action

- Advance the tube
- Inflate the balloon with 5 cc of normal saline
- If unsure that tube is properly placed, perform radiographic dye study to assure proper placement

Resources

Foltin G, Tunik M, Cooper A, et al. *Teaching Resource for Instructors in Prehospital Pediatrics.* The Center for Pediatric Emergency Medicine: New York; 2002.

Utah Department of Health, Bureau of Emergency Medical Services. http://hlunix.hl.state.ut.us/ems/

Children with Special Health Care Needs: Technology Assisted Children. EMSC National Clearinghouse; 1998. Book available from http://www.emsc.org/products/frameproducts.htm. Accessed June 2004.

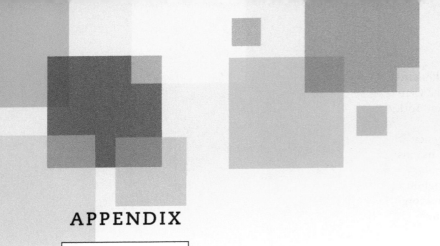

APPENDIX

A Problems and Solutions

Table A1. Medical Devices: Common Problems and Solutions		
Device	**Problem**	**Action**
Tracheostomy	Obstruction	Attempt assisted ventilation with high-concentration oxygen Attempt to suction Change tracheostomy tube Ventilate through stoma Transport
Tracheostomy	Dislodged	Replace tracheostomy Provide assisted ventilation with high-concentration oxygen through the stoma Transport
	Unable to reinsert	Attempt to place a tracheostomy tube one size smaller If attempt fails—attempt to place a similar size endotracheal tube If attempt fails—provide assisted ventilation through stoma or through the child's mouth while blocking the stoma
Home Ventilator	Respiratory Distress	Ask parents to check whether ventilator is functioning properly Assist in adjustment of ventilator Assess tracheostomy for obstruction Remove patient from ventilator and provide assisted ventilation
Pacemaker	Failure	Assess heart rate and perfusion Treat for shock Follow appropriate PALS guidelines Transport

continues

Table A1. Medical Devices: Common Problems and Solutions *(continued)*

Device	Problem	Action
Central Intravenous Catheter	Dislodged or damaged	Apply direct pressure to stop bleeding Clamp or tie exposed catheter to prevent further blood loss Assess and treat patient for hemothorax and shock Transport
Central Venous Catheter	Air embolism	Clamp the line Place patient on left side with head down Administer high-flow oxygen Transport
Central Venous Catheter Site	Signs of infection at the site	Treat as a potentially serious infection Transport
Oral or Nasal Feeding Catheter	Dislodged	Remove catheter Have patient seek medical attention for tube reinsertion
Surgically Placed Feeding Catheter	Dislodged	Cover open stoma with gauze Transport promptly
	Abdominal distension or obstruction	Unclamp tube Decompress stomach (aspirate air/fluids) Transport
CSF Shunt	Failure or obstruction	Treat ABCs Keep head elevated Give anticonvulsants for seizure activity Follow appropriate PALS guidelines for arrhythmias

Modified from: Foltin G, Tunik M, Cooper A, et al. *Teaching Resource for Instructors in Prehospital Pediatrics*. The Center for Pediatric Emergency Medicine: New York; 2002.

Resources

Utah Department of Health, Bureau of Emergency Medical Services. http://hlunix.hl.state.ut.us/ems/.
Children with Special Health Care Needs: Technology Assisted Children, 1998. EMSC National Clearinghouse.
    Available at: http://www.ems-c.org/products/frameproducts.htm. Accessed June 2004.

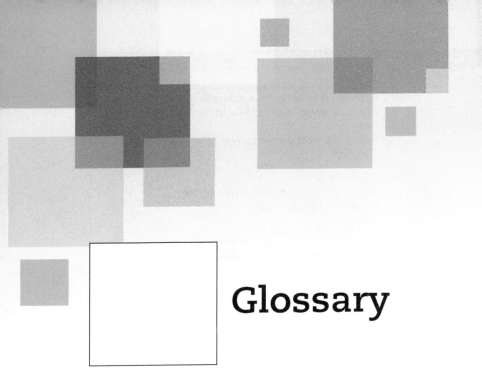

Glossary

absence (petite mal) seizures This type of seizure is characterized by brief loss of or change in consciousness, and is occasionally accompanied by loss of motor control.

acquired cerebral palsy Cerebral palsy resulting from brain damage that occurs in the first few months to years of life. It can occur from infections (e.g., meningitis) or injury (e.g., motor vehicle crash injury or other traumatic brain injury).

acquired immune deficiency syndrome (AIDS) A severe immunological disorder caused by the Human Immunodeficiency Virus (HIV). An HIV-positive person receives an AIDS diagnosis after developing one of the CDC-defined AIDS indicator illnesses. An HIV-positive person can also receive an AIDS diagnosis on the basis of certain blood tests (CD4 counts) and may not have experienced any serious illnesses. Over time, infection with HIV can weaken the immune system to the point that the system has difficulty fighting off certain opportunistic infections. (*Source:* Centers for Disease Control [CDC])

acute or chronic myelogenous leukemia (AML) Also called granulocytic, myelocytic, myeloblastic, or myeloid leukemia. A cancer of the blood in which too many immature myeloid cells (myeloblasts) are produced in the marrow and do not mature correctly, causing immune deficiency.

acyanotic defects Congenital abnormalities that do not cause cyanosis. These are generally septal defects, obstructions to the flow of blood, and incomplete heart development.

aortic stenosis An obstruction of blood flow across the aortic valve. A normal valve has three cusps, but a stenotic valve may have only one cusp (unicuspid) or two cusps (bicuspid), which are thick and stiff. It presents with varying degrees of severity and may require surgery to fix.

aplastic crisis Occurs in children with sick cell disease when the bone marrow stops producing red blood cells. Patients may appear pale, tired, and lethargic. Often requires a blood transfusion.

ascites An abnormal accumulation of fluid in the abdomen. It can occur due to trauma, chronic disease such as liver disease, or acute conditions such as appendicitis.

assist control mode A ventilator setting that allows a patient to initiate spontaneous breaths between the machine's delivered breaths.

asthma A respiratory disease characterized by shortness of breath and difficulty breathing due to a spasmodic contraction of the bronchi and accompanied by a wheezing sound.

asthma attack Recurrence of an episode of asthma.

ataxic cerebral palsy This rare form of cerebral palsy affects the sense of balance and depth perception causing poor coordination, muscle tremors, and an unsteady or wide-based gait.

atlantoaxial subluxation An instability of the first and second vertebrae in the neck. The lack of stability can cause compression of the spinal cord that can result in pain or paralysis. It is seen in a small percentage of children with Down syndrome.

atrial septal defect (ASD)   A hole in the septum separating the left and right atrium of the heart.

atrioventricular septal defect (AVSD)   Also called atrioventricular canal defect, results from a lack of separation of the atria and the ventricles into separate chambers, and a lack of separation of the mitral and tricuspid valves into two separate valves. Also described as a hole in the middle of the heart.

autosomal recessive disorder   Disorders caused by an error or mutation in a single unit of the genetic information. An autosomal disorder that is recessive can be expressed in a person only if both copies of the gene are altered. Examples of autosomal recessive disorder include cystic fibrosis and Tay-Sachs disease.

balloon arterial septostomy   A procedure performed during cardiac catherization. It enlarges the atrial opening to allow mixing of oxygenated with unoxygenated blood. In the past it was a palliative treatment for transposition of the great arteries and is still used as a treatment in patients with mitral, pulmonary, or tricuspid atresia.

balloon valvuloplasty   A procedure performed as part of a cardiac catheterization in which a narrowed heart valve is stretched open by threading flexible, sterile tubes into the inside of the heart, usually through the groin area. Used to repair conditions like pulmonary stenosis without open heart surgery.

biliary cirrhosis   A chronic liver disease that slowly destroys the bile ducts in the liver leading to diminished liver function and cirrhosis. The cause is unknown but linked to heredity.

biliary obstruction   Blockage of the bile duct that results in bile accumulating in the liver, elevating bilirubin levels in the bloodstream and causing jaundice. Can occur due to stones, duct inflammation, tumors, pancreatic swelling, cysts, or trauma.

BiPAP ventilatory support system   A machine that augments breathing by delivering pressurized air to keep the upper airway open. This is done through a mask attached to the face that senses a patient's breathing effort and then delivers the air through the mask when breathing in and out.

bradycardia   An abnormally slow heart rhythm.

bronchopulmonary dysplasia (BPD)   A chronic pulmonary disorder that typically occurs in premature infants as a result of lung-damage-caused oxygen toxicity or barotrauma from mechanical ventilation.

cardiac catherization   A diagnostic procedure to determine whether narrowing or blockages are present in the coronary arteries, and to measure heart valves and heart muscle function. Several specialized procedures are also performed. The procedure involves threading a catheter to the heart using a contrast medium such as a dye.

cardiomyopathy   A disease of the heart muscle where the heart loses its ability to pump blood, leading to irregular heartbeats or arrhythmias.

cerebral palsy (CP)   A medical condition caused by a permanent brain injury that occurs before, during, or shortly after birth. The effect of cerebral palsy is characterized by lack of muscle control and body movement. While it is not a progressive disease of the brain, the effects of cerebral palsy may change gradually over the years.

cerebral spinal fluid (CSF) shunt   A catheter placed to drain excess CSF fluid. The shunt is positioned to enable the CSF to be drained from the cerebral ventricles or subarachnoid spaces into another absorption site, the right atrium of the heart or, more commonly, the peritoneal cavity, through a catheter.

coarctation of the aorta   Narrowing of the aorta just past the point where the aorta and the subclavian artery meet.

congenital cardiovascular defects   A congenital cardiovascular defect occurs when the heart or blood vessels near the heart do not develop normally before birth. They occur in approximately 1% of newborns and are the most common congenital malformations (AHA).

congenital cerebral palsy   Cerebral palsy that is present at birth and not acquired after birth.

continuous positive airway pressure (CPAP)   Constant airway pressure delivered by a CPAP machine through a mask covering the mouth and/or nose in order to keep the alveoli from collapsing and allowing adequate respirations.

cor pulmonale   Also called right-sided heart failure. An alteration in the structure and function of the right ventricle caused by a primary disorder of the respiratory system.

cuffed tracheostomy tubes   A tracheostomy tube with an inflatable cuff on the distal end that, when inflated, eliminates or reduces air leaks as well as prevents aspiration.

Cushing's triad   A term used to describe signs and symptoms of increased intracranial pressure: (1) hypertension, (2) bradycardia, and (3) irregular respirations.

cystic fibrosis (CF)   An inherited disease that mainly affects the lungs and digestive system. In the lungs, a build-up of thick mucus makes it difficult to clear bacteria, leading to infection and inflammation. In the digestive tract, digestion and absorption are affected, and thick mucus blocks the ducts of the pancreas, preventing enzymes from reaching the intestines to digest food.

decannulation plug   A cap that is placed over the external opening of a fenestrated tracheostomy tube in order to completely redirect airflow into the upper airway.

developmental delay   A delay in a child's ability to meet age-appropriate growth and behaviors that usually results from prematurity or a prolonged illness; these children generally have the capability to eventually progress normally with their growth and development.

diabetes A condition characterized by high blood sugar resulting from the body's inability to use sugar (glucose) efficiently. In type 1 diabetes, the pancreas is not able to make enough insulin; in type 2 diabetes, the body is resistant to the effects of available insulin.

double cannula A removable inner cannula that fits inside a tracheostomy tube's outer cannula that provides a passageway for airflow and removal of secretions.

Down syndrome (DS) A congenital abnormality resulting from an extra chromosome (21) in the child's DNA that results in varying degrees of mental retardation and has distinct physical characteristics such as flattened occiput; slanted eyes; low set ears; large, protruding tongue; and short, broad hands with stubby fingers.

ductus A communication, channel, or opening between two structures.

ductus arteriosus An embryonic channel that connects the main pulmonary artery and the aorta of the dutus. Failure of the channel to close after birth results in a persistent communication between these two structures.

ductus venosus A venous channel that carries most of the placental venous flow into the heart through a connection between the left umbilical vein and the inferior vena cava. A persistent opening of the embryonic channel results in an abnormal pulmonary venous connection.

dyskinetic or athetoid cerebral palsy A form of cerebral palsy that is characterized by uncontrolled, slow movements.

encephalitis Inflammation of the brain.

endoscopic dilatation The stretching of the inside of a hollow organ or cavity using a lighted tube as a guide.

endoscopically placed feeding catheters Gastrostomy tubes that are placed surgically or percutaneously under the guidance of an endoscope. An endoscope is a tube-like instrument placed through a patient's mouth down the esophagus and into the stomach. A hole is then placed through the abdominal wall and into the stomach, guided by the endoscope.

esophageal varices Dilation of the veins in the esophagus resulting in an increased risk for esophageal bleeding or hemorrhage.

expiratory (EPAP) levels The amount of pressure that needs to be created for adequate exhalation when a patient inhales is measured as an EPAP level.

fenestrated tracheostomy tubes An opening or window in the upper curve of the tracheostomy tube that redirects air into the upper airway (the larynx) while allowing the child to speak and breathe through the nose and mouth.

Foley catheter Flexible plastic tube (catheter) inserted into the bladder to provide continuous urinary drainage.

foramen ovale An opening between the two atria of the heart in the fetus that generally closes shortly before or during birth but in rare instances may remain open resulting in a cardiac defect.

gastroesophageal reflux A backflow of gastric contents originating in the stomach and regurgitating up into the esophagus.

generator A machine that produces electricity.

G-tube button A type of feeding tube that is inserted into the stomach through the abdominal wall where the outside portion closes at the abdominal wall.

hemophilia A condition resulting in the inability of a person, generally males, to clot blood due to a missing or low supply of one of the factors required for normal blood clotting.

hepatomegaly Enlargement of the liver.

hydrocephalus An excessive buildup of cerebral spinal fluid in the ventricles of the brain.

hypoplastic left heart syndrome (HLHS) Underdevelopment of the left side of the heart, especially the left ventricle, which severely limits the ability of the left side of the heart to maintain adequate circulation throughout the body.

implanted vascular access port The reservoir, or access port, of a central venous catheter is implanted beneath the skin in a subcutaneous pocket. A special needle is often needed to gain access to this type of catheter.

indomethacin A drug used primarily for rheumatoid arthritis or degenerative joint disease that has anti-inflammatory, anagelsic, and antipyretic properties.

inspiratory (IPAP) levels The amount of pressure that needs to be created for adequate inhalation when a patient inhales is measured as an IPAP level.

internal cardiac defibrillator (ICD) A device inserted in the body that is designed to recognize certain types of abnormal heart rhythms (arrhythmias) and correct them by delivering timed electrical shocks, when needed, in order to restore a normal heart rhythm.

Kaposi's sarcoma A malignant abnormal tissue formation of the skin that is more commonly seen in acquired immune deficiency syndromes.

kyphoscoliosis Curvature of the spine that is both backward and lateral with an associated anteroposterior hump.

leads Wires from the pads placed on the patient's chest that lead to either a cardiac monitor, defibrillator, or wires associated with an internal pacemaker.

left-to-right shunts A term that is used to denote blood flow from the left side of the heart where there is higher pressure through a defect to the right side of the heart.

leukemia Uncontrolled rapid abnormal growth of blood cells resulting in nonfunctioning cells in the blood or bone marrow.

ligation Binding or tying together tissue or a vessel with a band or thread in order to constrict or close it.

malacia Abnormal softening of an organ or of tissues themselves.

mental retardation Below normal intellectual function that occurs during a child's developmental period resulting in an impairment of the ability to adapt to his or her environment.

MIC-Key A type of feeding tube whose internal end is usually placed in the stomach and the external portion is outside the abdominal wall. The tube extends several inches past the abdominal wall and can be directly accessed and hooked up to a bag with liquid nutrients.

mitral Pertaining to the bicuspid or mitral valve in the heart.

muscular dystrophy Atrophy and wasting away of muscles that result from a flaw in muscle protein genes that may or may not be inherited.

myelomeningocele A defect occurring early in utero where a portion of the spinal cord and associated membranes abnormally protrude through a gap in the spine.

myoclonic seizures A type of seizure activity characterized by sudden startle-like episodes where the body flexes or briefly extends.

nasal continuous positive airway pressure (CPAP) Steady flow of air given through a ventilator. Prevents collapse of the airway and increases oxygen to the body.

nasogastric uube (NGT) A tube placed through the nose that extends to the stomach for delivery of medications and/or nutrition for digestion. This type of feeding type is usually placed for short-term use.

nasojejunal tube (NJT) A tube placed through the nose and then threaded through the pyloric sphincter of the stomach into the small bowel through to the jejunum. This is usually placed by a radiologist under fluoroscopy.

neurologic diseases Diseases related to the brain or neurological system (for example, autism in children and Alzheimer's disease in adults).

nontunneled central venous catheters A central venous catheter that is inserted directly into a vein and then advanced into the superior vena cava. This type of central venous catheter is not usually surgically placed.

obstructive lesions Generally refers to congenital cardiac lesions that block the flow of blood. An example is pulmonic stenosis where the pulmonary artery is small, so the flow of blood from the right ventricle through the pulmonary artery is decreased due to the small size of the artery.

obturator A flexible plastic stylet with a rounded tip that is inserted into a tracheostomy tube to prevent kinking and to guide the tube through the tracheostomy stoma during tube insertion.

orogastric tube (G-tube) A feeding tube placed through the mouth into the stomach. Usually used in neonates.

osteogenesis imperfecta (OI) Autosomal dominant disorder of connective tissue characterized by brittle bones that fracture easily (also called brittle bone disease).

pancreatic insufficiency Pancreatic insufficiency occurs when the pancreas does not secrete enough chemicals and digestive enzymes for normal digestion to occur.

percutaneous endoscopic gastrostomy (PEG) A procedure for placing a feeding tube without having to perform an open operation on the abdomen (laparotomy). A gastrostomy (a surgical opening into the stomach) is made percutaneously (through the skin) using an endoscope (a flexible, lighted instrument) to determine where to place the feeding tube in the stomach and to secure it in place.

peripherally inserted central venous catheter (PICC) A nontunneled central venous catheter that is usually inserted directly into the basilic or cephalic vein of the arm for the purpose of shorter-term venous access.

placenta Special tissue that joins the mother and fetus to provide hormones necessary for a successful pregnancy, and supplies the fetus with water and nutrients (food) from the mother's blood.

pressure-cycled ventilators A machine that mechanically delivers a preset pressure of air with each breath to a child who is unable to ventilate independently.

prostaglandins A class of naturally occurring chemicals that are made in many tissues of the body. They (among other chemicals) contribute to proper functioning of the stomach and intestinal lining, the platelets, and the kidneys. Prostaglandin E is used in the postnatal period as a medication to keep the ductus arteriosus open in newborns with complex congenital heart disease, whereby the flow of blood is decreased or blocked entirely between the two sides of the heart. The ductus arteriosis is a connection between the two sides of the heart used during fetal life that closes the first few days of life. In some heart conditions this connection must stay open to sustain life until a surgical procedure can be performed on the infant to allow mixing of blood.

pulmonary atresia Small or undeveloped pulmonary valve, which results in an inability to pump blood to the lungs from the right ventricle through the pulmonary artery.

pulmonary stenosis Abnormal narrowing of the opening into the pulmonary artery from the right ventricle.

racemic epinephrine There are two isomers of epinephrine; racemic epinephrine is one form. It is a medication that is usually nebulized and is sometimes used in small children with croup or bronchiolitis.

rectal prolapse   The abnormal movement of the rectal mucosa down to or through the anal opening.

respiratory distress syndrome   A condition (mostly of premature infants) due to insufficient surfactant in the lungs with results in the inability of the air sacs to stay open.

sepsis   The presence of organisms (usually bacteria) in the bloodstream or tissues. This can be a life-threatening condition when accompanied by shock.

sick sinus syndrome   A disorder in the heart's sinus node that affects how heartbeats are generated and how they are conducted. It usually causes a slow heart rate.

sickle cell anemia   An inherited autosomal recessive disorder that causes abnormal hemoglobin in blood cells, leading to infections and organ damage. Red blood cells appear "sickled."

single cannula   A tracheostomy tube that is one tube. Provides a single passage for airflow and suctioning of secretions.

sinus arrythmia   Slight variation in cycling of the sinus rhythm, usually one that exceeds 0.12 seconds between the longest and shortest cycles. Sinus arrhythmia is a normal finding in children and young adults and tends to diminish or disappear with age.

sinus tachycardia   Heart rhythm that originates in the sinus node and proceeds through the rest of the electrical conduction system, but is faster than normal.

spastic cerebral palsy   Common type of CP where children have stiff and jerky movements. They often have a hard time moving from one position to another and holding and letting go of objects.

spina bifida   A birth defect in which the neural tube fails to close during fetal development and a portion of the spinal cord and nerves fails to develop properly.

splenic sequestration crisis   Occurs in young children with sickle cell disease when a large portion of the child's blood volume becomes trapped in the spleen. Early signs include paleness, an enlarged spleen, and pain in the abdomen.

splenomegaly   Enlargement of the spleen.

stent   A device implanted in a vessel used to help keep it open.

supraventricular tachycardia   A series of rapid heartbeats arising from the upper chambers of the heart that can cause the heart to beat very rapidly or erratically and may lead to inadequate blood supplies to the body.

synchronized intermittent mechanical ventilation (SIMV)   A ventilator mode that allows a patient to spontaneously breathe, without ventilator assistance, between the machine-delivered breaths by synchronizing the ventilator's breath with the patient's breathing effort.

tet spells   Seen in infants with tetralogy of Fallot where they develop episodes of bluish skin from crying or feeding.

tetralogy of Fallot   A congenital heart disease consisting of four defects: a ventricular septal defect, an enlargement of the right ventricle, pulmonic valve stenosis or narrowing, and an overriding aorta.

tonic-clonic (grand mal) seizures   Usually characterized by muscle rigidity, violent rhythmic muscle contractions, and loss of conciousness. The condition is caused by abnormal electrical activity in the nerve cells of the brain.

trachea decannulation   Permanent removal of the tracheal tube.

tracheal atresia   A congenital absence of or maldevelopment of the trachea.

tracheal stenosis   Narrowing of the tracheal lumen (can be congenital or acquired).

tracheoesophageal fistula   A condition where a fistula connects the trachea and esophagus.

tracheomalacia   Abnormal collapse of the tracheal walls.

tracheostomy   A surgical opening in the neck that creates a stoma between the trachea and anterior surface of the neck to aid in the passage of air.

transposition of the great arteries   A congenital heart defect involving abnormal development of the great arteries (the aorta and the pulmonary artery) during the time the heart is forming prior to birth. The aorta ends up being connected to the right ventricle, and the pulmonary artery is connected to the left ventricle, which is the opposite of how they are normally connected.

tricuspid atresia   A congenital heart defect in which the tricuspid valve and right ventricle do not develop properly, preventing oxygen-poor (blue) blood from reaching the lungs via its normal pathway.

tricuspid valve   The heart valve that controls blood flow from the right atrium into the right ventricle.

truncus arteriosus   A congenital heart defect involving incomplete separation of the great arteries (the aorta and the pulmonary artery) during the time the heart is forming prior to birth.

tunneled central venous catheters   A central venous catheter that goes through the skin and then is advanced through subcutaneous tissue until it is inserted into the appropriate vein for further advancement to the superior vena cava. This type of catheter is usually surgically placed.

Turner's syndrome   A genetic disorder affecting only females whereby there is only one X chromosome or one of the two X chromosomes is damaged.

type 1 diabetes   Previously known as insulin-dependent diabetes mellitus (IDDM) or juvenile diabetes. The pancreas stops making insulin. Type 1 diabetes usually begins before the age of 30.

type 2 diabetes   Previously known as noninsulin-dependent diabetes mellitus (NIDDM) or adult-onset diabetes. A condition in which the body either makes too little insulin or cannot use the insulin it makes to use blood glucose as energy, which can often be controlled through meal plans, physical activity plans, medication, or insulin.

vagal nerve stimulator (VNS)   A small generator that sends electrical activity to the brain to prevent seizures. It is surgically implanted into the chest, under the collarbone and attached to the left vagus nerve. A magnet external to the chest is used to activate it.

vagus nerve   The tenth cranial nerve that has both motor and sensory function.

vascular rings   A congenital condition where the great vessels abnormally surround the trachea. These vessels can potentially cause compression of the trachea, causing respiratory symptoms. Surgery is the treatment for this condition.

ventricular septal defect   An abnormal opening in the wall between the right and left ventricles.

ventricular tachycardia   A condition in which the ventricles cause a very fast heartbeat.

ventriculoatrial shunt   A type of CSF shunt that is a catheter used to drain fluid from the cerebral ventricle into the right atrium of the heart.

ventriculoperitoneal shunt   A type of CSF shunt that is a catheter used to drain fluid from the ventricles in the brain into the peritoneum.

volume ventilators   A machine that delivers a fixed tidal volume of air with each breath to a child who is unable to adequately independently ventilate.

Wolff-Parkinson-White   A condition caused by an extra (or accessory) pathway from the atria to the ventricles, which leads to rapid heart beats (supraventricular tachycardia) and symptomatically causes palpitations.

Index

traumatic brain injuries, 27
traumatically disabled children, 26–28
tricuspid atresia, 18
tricuspid valve, 13, 19
trisomy 21, 23
truncus arteriosus, 19
tuberculosis, pulmonary, 42

upper respiratory infection (URI), 8
urinary incontinence, 24, 34
urinary tract infection (UTI), 33
URI (upper respiratory infection), 8
UTIs (urinary tract infections), 33

vagal nerve stimulators (VNS), 31, 81–82
vagus nerve, 81–82
valium, 35
vascular access ports
    central venous catheters, 66
    comparisons, 67
    implanted, 66–67
vaso-occlusive crisis, 38, 41
venous catheter occlusion, 87

ventilator-dependent children, 62
ventilators. *see also* home ventilators; mechanical
    ventilation
for quadriplegic children, 27
ventricular peritoneal shunt (VP shunt), 27
ventricular septal defect (VSD), 11, 13, 16, 19
ventricular tachycardia (VT), 20
ventriculoatrial (VA) shunts, 79
ventriculoperitoneal (VP) shunt, 31, 79
verbal support, 51
vital signs
    baseline, 52
    "normal," 52
VNS (vagal nerve stimulators), 31, 81–82
volume ventilators, 60
VSD (ventricular septal defect), 11, 13, 16, 19
VT (ventricular tachycardia), 20

WBCs (white blood cells), 39–40
wheelchairs, 27, 48
wheezing, 4, 8
white blood cells (WBCs), 39–40
Wolff-Parkinson-White (WPW) syndrome, 20

Additional Credits

Chapter 1
Figure 1-1 © Photodisc/Getty Images
Figure 1-2 Courtesy of Terry Adirim, MD

Chapter 3
Figure 3-1 © Stock Connection Distribution/Alamy Images

Chapter 4
Figure 4-1 © Ken Sherman/Phototake

Chapter 5
Figure 5-3 © Tom Prettyman/PhotoEdit

Chapter 6
Figure 6-1 Courtesy of Terry Adirim, MD

Chapter 9
Figure 9-1 © Paul Whitehill/Alamy Images
Figure 9-2 © Michael Newman/PhotoEdit

Chapter 11
Figure 11-2 Courtesy of Smith Medical
Figure 11-5 Courtesy of Terry Adirim, MD
Figure 11-6 Reprinted by permission of Nellcor Puritan Bennett Inc., Pleasanton, California
Figure 11-7 Reprinted by permission of Nellcor Puritan Bennett Inc., Pleasanton, California

Chapter 12
Figure 12-1 Courtesy of Becton, Dickinson and Company

Photos have also been supplied by Jones and Bartlett Publishers.